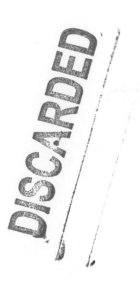
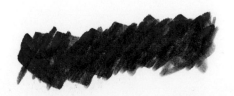

SLIMMER

SLIMMER

The New Mediterranean Way to Lose Weight

HARRY PAPAS

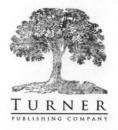

TURNER
PUBLISHING COMPANY

TURNER PUBLISHING COMPANY

200 4th Avenue North • Suite 950
Nashville, Tennessee 37219

445 Park Avenue • 9th Floor
New York, NY 10022

www.turnerpublishing.com

Slimmer: The New Mediterranean Way to Lose Weight

The weight-loss principles in this book are not intended to provide a cure, diagnosis, or treatment, nor are they a substitute for the advice of a physician. Before beginning any new health or weight-loss program, you should seek the advice of a doctor or other medical professional.

Cover design by Gina Binkley
Interior design by Glen Edelstein

Library of Congress Cataloging-in-Publication Data

Papadopoulos, Charilaos, 1970-
  Slimmer : the new Mediterranean way to lose weight / Harry Papas. -- 1st american ed.
    p. cm.
  ISBN 978-1-59652-856-7
  1. Reducing diets. 2. Weight loss. I. Title.
  RM222.2.P33 2012
  613.2'5--dc23

                          2011045158

Printed in the United States of America
12 13 14 15 16 17 18—0 9 8 7 6 5 4 3 2 1

First American Edition

Originally published in Athens, Greece as *Slimmer: The Mediterranean Way to Lose Weight* by Livani Publishing Organization.

To the wonderful people of the United States and especially to my excellent literary agent, Coleen O' Shea, the first person who paved the way for *Slimmer* to be given to American readers too.

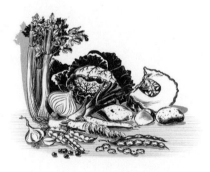

Contents

Acknowledgments

Some of the most important things in my life come from the USA: music, movies, style, education, and friends. For all these I am grateful. It is because of my gratitude that I offer my Slimmer program to help my friends in the United States who struggle with health and weight problems.

As a young man in Greece, a blessed Mediterranean country, I also used to have weight problems. When I found the solution, I wanted to share my discoveries and I wrote this book, which became an immediate bestseller in Greece. What I want now is to provide my friends in America and other countries around the world with my unique solution to health and weight issues.

In the process of creating this book, five important people helped me to accomplish it: my wonderful agent, Coleen O' Shea, of the Allen O'Shea Literary Agency, the creative writer Liz Scott, my visionary publisher, Todd Bottorff, and executive editor Diane Gedymin, and my lovely editor, Christina Huffines. I am very grateful to them for their help and support in bringing *Slimmer* to you.

SLIMMER

The Slimmer Story

In many ways, the Slimmer story is really my story. As a young man growing up in modern Athens, Greece, I had an enviable life. I looked good, felt good, was popular and smart, and saw nothing but continued success and happiness in my future. I ate a relatively healthy diet, without too many indulgences, and was physically fit and active. Then something changed.

Many people gain weight as they get older, particularly in middle age, because their diet does not reflect their change in lifestyle and the need to adjust to a natural slowing of the metabolism. But what happened to me, and what happens to millions of people around the world, can be more sudden and drastic and can occur at any stage in life regardless of age. Events such as divorce, job loss, family and romantic problems, depression, stress, and even boredom can create a weight-gain cycle that quickly and easily spins out of control. Before we know it, we are looking in the mirror at someone we no longer recognize.

For me, my entry into a new academic environment at college

proved to be the trigger for the unraveling of my good health. I was now merely a small fish in a very big pond. No one envied me. In fact no one even knew me. I was stressed, depressed, lonely, and bored, not only with my uninspiring choice of economics as a major but with my daily, unrewarding routine. In a very short time my life had gone from a sunny romantic fairy tale to a gloomy Shakespearean tragedy and in the process, food became my only friend. I reached for junk food for comfort and chocolate for fulfillment. My daily calorie and fat intake snowballed as I ate more and more of these empty calories at every turn. I felt sluggish and unable to break from the sedentary existence I had created for myself. In one year I gained 110 pounds.

Unhappy and unhealthy, I knew I needed to lose weight. So I began dieting. If one diet didn't work for me I'd try a different one from the multitude available. I'd lose a little bit of weight and then quickly gain it back. Or I'd find a particular diet difficult to stick with and not lose any weight at all. Often the food was tasteless and unsatisfying, or the ingredients were too unusual and hard to find. Sometimes the strictness of a program itself would make me feel so deprived and full of cravings that I would abandon it in a moment of weakness and head for the nearest pizzeria. Surely there had to be a better and easier way.

I made a decision. At the University of Athens I switched my major from Economics to Diet and Nutrition. If there was a better way, I would figure it out myself! As a Diet and Nutrition major, I was exposed to a great deal of valuable research including the landmark 1960s Seven Countries Study which was, in many ways, responsible for the popularity of the Mediterranean diet. The results determined that the Mediterranean diet eaten in Greece and specifically on the island of Crete was the healthiest for reducing heart attacks and coronary disease (more on this study in Chapter 1). And since then, the components of the traditional Mediterranean diet, including olive oil, lean protein, whole grains, and lots of fresh fruit and vegetables, have been determined to be beneficial for a number of health issues we are facing in today's world including diabetes, metabolic syndrome, arthritis, depression, and yes—obesity and the need for healthy weight loss. Here in my own country, the answer, at least in part, was right in front of me. But there was more.

Research was showing that psychological and emotional support, stress-free living, and a return to the basics of everyday life can have an enormous effect on the success of one's quest for better health, including the journey towards a healthy weight. Not surprisingly, the true Mediterranean diet that had been part of the 1960s study had contained this vital component as well. Life was simpler then. Family and good friends were naturally a part of the enjoyment of good food and provided us with a healthy connection with others on a regular basis. Availability dictated the menu which was always fresh, local, and affordable. People were outdoors in the sun more, not hidden behind computer screens in office cubicles.

Much has changed, even in the Mediterranean countries, in the decades since the study, with the rapid growth of high technology that has allowed for instant everything, from Internet messaging to microwave French fries. With all that we were gaining (including weight!) we were losing so much more. Surely this lifestyle element had to be an integral piece of the weight-loss puzzle too. The simple, traditional Mediterranean existence, so envied and romanticized by people around the globe, needed to be tapped into as a vital element for success. What could be better than actually "slimming" down eating delicious, fresh food in the good company of friends and family while enjoying and appreciating the natural beauty and simple pleasures of the world around us?

And so, I gathered together what I believed were the central components needed for a healthy approach to not only losing weight, but living a life that was full and rewarding. I took the healthy ingredients of the authentic Mediterranean diet and lifestyle, combined it with the needs of the modern dieter, such as ease of preparation and portability, and incorporated new conclusions from research in the diet and nutrition field such as adding extra fat-burning ingredients and following newer recommendations for daily nutrition. In this way, the diet I created was truly unique. Never before had the Mediterranean diet, specifically the southern Greek diet, been revised along the lines of modern science and nutrition. This approach proved to be the vital difference between all other Mediterranean weight-loss approaches, and the one that helped create success for so many people and which will now help you find and reach your ideal weight.

Perhaps most important, I made sure that every single recipe was not only just somewhat tasty, but remarkably delicious. They are Greek recipes made even better, many of which have been enjoyed by both local and celebrity visitors to my mother and aunt's restaurant in Cefalonia. As a fussy eater, I knew just how important this aspect of appealing and satisfying meals would be.

The result was Slimmer, the program that is about to change your life. It has already changed the lives of millions of Greek dieters and I know it will change yours. You'll not only become "slimmer" as I did, but you will finally be free of the obstacles that have stood in the way of the "slimmer" you and the happier and healthier life you deserve.

Today I am a registered dietician specializing in overweight and obesity issues. I have established a leading health and diet center in Greece and have led support groups to help dieters who are struggling to navigate the problems we all face when weight gain becomes a terrifying reality in our lives. For the past 12 years I have seen Slimmer work its magic on so many people and have been witness to the astounding transformations that occur. Be part of the magic and watch your life change before your eyes.

Welcome to *Slimmer: The New Mediterranean Way to Lose Weight*.

Harry Papas, ATHENS, JULY 2011

PART ONE

THE SLIMMER NUTRITIONAL PROGRAM

Chapter 1

Slimmer and the Mediterranean Diet and Lifestyle

Studies continue to show that following a Mediterranean-style diet, which incorporates the traditional foods of the Mediterranean regions of Greece and parts of France and Italy, is beneficial to our health on a number of levels. From lowering the risk for heart attack and stroke, to warding off cognitive impairment as well as Type 2 diabetes, cancer, and even obesity, the benefits are numerous and impressive. But what exactly defines a Mediterranean diet and can it form the nucleus of a successful weight-loss program?

The important 1960s Seven Countries Study, conceived and carried out by the American nutritionist Ancel Keys in conjunction with the University of Minnesota, aimed to examine the diet and coronary health of approximately 13,000 men ages 40 to 59, located in seven different countries (Italy, Greece, former Yugoslavia, the Netherlands, Finland, United States, and Japan). Unique for its time, the study was the first to explore the association between diet and the risk of disease among contrasting populations. The results were nothing less than groundbreaking and would fashion our modern view of healthy eating for decades to come.

Interestingly, it was found that the southern Greek population, specifically on the island of Crete, were the least likely to develop coronary disease. Remarkably, the premature death rate from heart attack for Greek men was 90 percent lower than that of American men! Elevated factors that contributed to the risk of heart attack such as high blood cholesterol levels, high blood pressure, and obesity, were much lower for those consuming a Mediterranean diet than for those eating a northern European or American-style diet.

The decades following this monumental study have borne out the same results. Study after study has shown how healthy the traditional Mediterranean diet and lifestyle can be, particularly in combatting today's ever-growing health issues of obesity, diabetes, and heart disease, collectively known as metabolic syndrome.

What did the Mediterranean diet consist of, according to the Seven Countries Study? It was primarily plant based with an emphasis on fresh vegetables and fruits, whole grains, lean protein (mostly from fish), olive oil, and moderate amounts of wine. Dairy products, including cheese and yogurt, were plentiful and eaten often, while red meat, poultry, and eggs, which were less readily available, were eaten less frequently. Processed foods were virtually unheard of and sweets of any kind were definitely enjoyed in very small portions. As is still often practiced today, the largest meal was eaten at lunchtime, with a brief period of rest afterwards before heading back to work. In the evening, light suppers were the norm. Snacking was almost nonexistent.

By comparison, the diet consumed by northern European participants and Americans consisted of much larger amounts of animal protein, saturated fat, and refined carbohydrates such as white bread and processed cereals. In part due to the technological advances made in manufacturing, mass-produced "foods" which offered extreme ease of preparation and were budget-friendly, became

Japan and the Seven Countries Study

Today Japan enjoys the longest life expectancy of any country. In fact during the Seven Countries Study, both Japan and the Greek Islands had a low incidence of coronary disease and low levels of serum cholesterol, but for Japan there was a catch. Due to the high levels of sodium intake, stress, and cigarette smoking, the Japanese were fighting a losing battle against high blood pressure and an extremely elevated risk of stroke. In spite of their otherwise healthy diet of low-fat, low animal protein, and healthy carbohydrates, the Japanese were considered to be in need of a somewhat better diet and a much better lifestyle approach.

Oddly, in the past decades as Western diet trends have become popular, the Japanese risk of stroke has decreased but the incidence of obesity and heart disease has risen. Blood pressure may be down, but cholesterol levels are definitely up. The exception to this trend is the Japanese population followed since 1975 and written about in the Okinawa Centenarian Study, who are considered today to be the healthiest and longest living population in the world. Their active and fulfilling lives as well as their healthy diet habits seem to be the keys to their well-being and longevity.

popularly accepted and consumed. In exchange for this convenience—including longer shelf-life with the addition of preservatives—quality, freshness, and the healthfulness of local sustenance were sacrificed.

The modern diet of the Mediterranean, although in many ways still probably healthier than the average American diet, has been adversely affected by technology and globalization too. Processed foods and fast-food restaurants are more readily found and the stress of faster-paced living has taken its toll. Obesity is a concern in many areas of the Mediterranean due in part to the importation of Western foods and eating habits. Sadly, even a good amount of Mediterranean eaters have strayed from the traditional, and need to return to a healthier approach to cooking and eating. However, many Mediterranean eaters still have diets similar to those of their predecessors and thus reap the same benefits.

In addition to the Mediterranean population's traditional diet, the lifestyle of the people in these regions was also of great significance in the Seven Countries Study. Unscathed by the pressures of modern life, Mediterranean residents at that time enjoyed an existence that was physically active, emotionally grounded, pleasurable, and rewarding due to simple approaches to work, family, friends, and life in general. Compared to the American lifestyle of escalated stress and anxiety coupled with a sedentary existence, the southern Greek population was far better off in terms of health and most likely, far happier and more contented as well.

It is now fifty years after the Seven Countries Study was initially conducted, and although we can't go back to pre-1960s Greece, we can certainly try to re-create the advantages that it had for good health and weight control. And we can do this by consuming healthful traditional ingredients and adopting, whenever possible, the admirable approach to life that was so significant to the well-being of the study's Mediterranean population.

We don't need to be a farmer on the island of Crete to benefit from what we know about living a healthy existence. We don't even need to be walking along the beach in southern Greece (although it would be fun to imagine!) in order to reap the benefits of the Mediterranean lifestyle. We simply need to learn how to eat more healthfully and live more rewardingly. And Slimmer is here to show you how.

THE MEDITERRANEAN DIET

Let's start by taking a closer look at some of the diet's traditional Mediterranean ingredients you will be enjoying on the Slimmer program, why they are significant for good health and weight loss, and how they are utilized in the Slimmer diet program.

The Power of Purslane

This weed of the succulent plant family has been both a medicinal and culinary wonder since ancient times and was a popular component of the traditional Mediterranean diet. Still eaten often in Greece and other areas of the Mediterranean, grass-fed animals often consumed good quantities of purslane as well, and in turn passed on its nutritional benefits in dairy and meat products. As one of the only plant sources of omega-3 fatty acids, in addition to flax seeds and walnuts, it is popular with vegetarian eaters and is occasionally found in ethnic markets in the United States. Deemed beneficial for problems such as arthritis, inflammation, respiratory ailments, and poor circulation, purslane makes an excellent addition to salads and omelettes. It is likely that the omega-3 in purslane along with that of Mediterranean fish consumption contributed, at least in part, to the healthy heart results of the Seven Countries Study.

Fresh Fruits and Vegetables

Having the luxury of picking fresh figs from a backyard tree to eat with freshly made goat cheese and local honey is something few Americans know. But in traditional Mediterranean populations, high quality, locally produced fresh fruit, vegetables, and other ingredients were commonly and readily available, free of unwanted chemical pesticides, and packed with nutrients from the rich, untainted soil. As a result, these plant-based foods carried fewer man-made toxins and a much higher level of vitamins and minerals. On the other hand, when we fly in fruits and vegetables from far-off locations, particularly those that have been treated with chemicals to preserve their appearance and are grown in acreage that has been depleted of its nutrients, we lose the powerhouse of nutrition that we would get if we consumed only locally grown, organic counterparts. Therefore, choosing farm-fresh, nontreated produce is the best and healthiest way to replicate the traditional Mediterranean diet's approach to fresh fruit and vegetables. And eating a good variety on a regular basis in order to provide an array of nutrition is recommended on the Slimmer program.

Certainly not all varieties of fresh produce are available to each of us year-round, but your goal should be to buy locally grown fruits and vegetables whenever possible and choose frozen or dried versions when necessary as a healthy alternative. Canned and processed fruits and their juices, in particular, can contain added unwanted sugar while canned vegetables often contain added unwanted sodium.

For weight loss, fiber-rich fruits and vegetables can ward off hunger pangs by keeping us satisfied for longer periods of time while increasing our metabolism so that we burn calories more efficiently. This is why you will see the inclusion of fruits such as prunes, kiwis, and other fiber-rich selections on each day's menu. You will also see the inclusion of fruits such as oranges, grapefruits, and other citrus varieties, for example, or the recommendation of red fruits such as raspberries and grapes, to ensure good intake of a variety of vitamins and minerals required for good health as you shed pounds. Too often dieters deprive themselves of these important micronutrients when reducing calories. Slimmer makes sure this does not occur.

Lean protein

Moderate amounts of lean protein were part of the traditional Mediterranean diet. For those living on the coast, fish was conveniently available and usually the protein of choice, while others living further inland may have opted for more poultry consumption and occasionally lean beef and lamb.

The key is that lean animal protein was most certainly secondary to the consumption of plant-based foods including whole grains, fruits, and vegetables. When fish was eaten, it was usually cold-water, omega-3-rich varieties such as salmon and sardines. Red meat, consumed infrequently due to lack of availability, was generally from grass-fed animals, resulting in much leaner cuts of meat and a higher nutritional value.

Poultry was generally farm raised and allowed to peck at seeds and insects, which indirectly provided increased omega-3 consumption while producing healthier, nutrient-rich chicken and eggs.

Today we can replicate these selections by opting for free-range chicken and meats from grass-fed animals, without hormones or added boosters for growth. Eggs from free-range chickens, enriched with omega-3, are good choices as well. Fish that is wild caught as opposed to farm raised varieties that may contain high levels of toxins is also the healthier choice, and as an added bonus usually contains higher levels of omega-3.

For weight-loss purposes, not only is lean protein a far better option than fattier varieties because of its lower saturated fat content, but it also has the ability to increase the body's lean muscle mass and fat-burning ability. Omega-3, in addition to all its other benefits, has been shown to reduce leptin levels, a hormone that when elevated is associated with obesity and which, when lowered, can increase metabolism and help the body burn calories more efficiently.

Whole grains

When many people think of a Mediterranean diet they immediately envision bowls of pasta and delicious breads and pizza. Although these are definitely a part of the Mediterranean menu, they are not consumed at the high levels that you might imagine and certainly not at the levels consumed in America. Pasta, beloved by every Italian and enjoyed throughout the Mediterranean, is usually served as a first course in quite small quantities as a prelude to the main meal which consists of a protein selection, vegetables, and a salad. When it appears as part of a main course, the portion size is very moderate.

Whole grains are, of course, found in many forms beyond flour in pasta and bread. Whole wheat kernels, farro, oats, brown rice, barley, buckwheat, and any number of other whole grains are often incorporated into stews and soups, and served as accompaniments to protein and vegetable selections, as well as in breakfast cereal form. These highly nutritious, less processed grains were and still are an integral part of the healthy Mediterranean diet. And fortunately today, the availability of even the more unusual whole grains is increasing in America. Many companies even offer organic versions.

A diet that is high in fiber can be a true boost to weight loss, and eating a variety of whole grains can offer you that advantage. Oat consumption in particular can help a dieter avoid highly fluctuating glucose levels in the blood, which will assist in keeping his or her mood and energy level on an even keel.

Dairy products

A somewhat surprising conclusion from the Seven Countries Study was the amount of dairy, including cheese and yogurt, which was regularly consumed by healthy participants. However, we need only think back to the phenomenon of the famous yogurt-eating centenarians of Russia and consider our current knowledge of probiotics—healthy bacteria—to see the connection. Assisting in regular digestion and helping to boost the immune system, probiotic-containing yogurt and other foods containing probiotics can certainly make a difference in the health of a population. Plain, unsweetened, strained Greek yogurt, only now gaining popularity in America, has been a mainstay of the Mediterranean diet for quite some time.

Cheese and milk, in moderation, have also been mainstays and although they may contribute saturated fat, the lower animal-protein consumption by those living in the region seems to counterbalance any detrimental effect the fats would otherwise have. In addition, the preference for olive oil over butter in cooking and eating has also limited the effect of what might otherwise have been considered a larger than acceptable amount of fat-laden dairy products.

When making choices today, adults should opt for reduced-fat and organic dairy whenever possible. Overly sugar-laden, dessert-like yogurts that bear little resemblance to the real thing should be exchanged for plain yogurts that can be made sweet by adding fresh fruit, honey, and even granola.

Dairy products rich in calcium can act as a metabolic trigger to weight loss. Research has shown that dieters who include milk and yogurt in their program can lose more weight than those who do not. Milk consumption can also help to keep insulin levels low. When elevated, particularly after a meal, high insulin can signal the body to hang on to its fat rather than burn it off.

Olive oil

The highlight of the Seven Countries Study was most certainly the olive oil consumption witnessed in the healthiest Mediterranean populations. Researchers concluded that it was no doubt the primary dietary element responsible for the reduced amount of coronary incidents seen, because of its effect on lowering cholesterol levels and keeping arteries healthy.

Olive oil, a healthful, plant-based oil, is high in nutrition and omega-9 (oleic acid), a monounsaturated fat. The extra-virgin type, which is made from the first pressing, is richest in antioxidant content and was used quite liberally in the traditional Mediterranean diet as a cooking fat as well as a flavoring oil for salads and vegetables. The olives were usually locally grown and pressed and had subtleties in flavor like a regional wine would have.

Today there are numerous brands and types of olive oil available in America from a number of countries as well as domestic varieties from within the United States. Organic oils are also seen and the selection available can range in price quite dramatically. Finding a pleasant tasting, affordable extra virgin olive oil you enjoy is the important factor and using it in moderation, when cooking and eating, will provide you with the numerous health benefits it offers.

As an alternative to butter, olive oil can provide a dieter with small hints of intense and satisfying flavor as well as a dose of nutrition in the form of antioxidants. Used sparingly during the Slimmer program and a bit more liberally during your maintenance, olive oil will add a wonderful aspect to your ultimate enjoyment of Mediterranean cuisine.

Wine and vinegar

Mediterraneans enjoy their wine and researchers in the Seven Countries Study concluded that it was a regular part of their healthy diet and one of the elements that helped to decrease the risk of heart disease. The amount consumed, however, was relatively small by comparison to Western alcohol consumption, and was almost exclusively reserved for accompanying a meal. Red wine in particular was often enjoyed in southern Greece as well as Crete.

We know today that wine contains an antioxidant known as resveratrol that has been touted for its ability to decrease heart disease, lower blood sugar, and even slow the aging process. Yet, resveratrol is also available to us in a number of other foods and drinks including red-skinned fruits and their juices, peanuts, and even chocolate. If you do not drink, don't begin. Despite the advantages of moderate alcohol consumption, there are also many health concerns that exist including increased risk of cancer, negative medication interactions, and alcohol dependence.

Vinegar, made through a further fermentation process from wine and other beverages, resulting in an alcohol-free condiment, is becoming viewed more and more as a healthy addition to the modern diet and was used often in the traditional Mediterranean diet as well. It has even been found in some studies that small amounts of vinegar (such as that used in a salad with olive oil) can help people to lose weight. This is also true of lemon juice, which is a traditional Mediterranean ingredient and is often recommended in Slimmer to be used on vegetables and with fish.

The way in which lemon and vinegar helps with weight loss is actually twofold:

1. The inclusion of an acid such as acetic or citric acid at a meal can reduce the quick effect that highly refined carbohydrate foods can have on digestion, and hence, blood glucose levels. By reducing this impact, dieters feel satiated longer and are less likely to submit to snack cravings from hunger or dips in energy.

2. Adding these types of acid to the diet has been shown to help burn one's intake of fat. A recent Japanese study showed that mice fed a high-fat diet, but who ingested small amounts of vinegar as well, were less fat than those who did not receive the acid supplementation but ate the same high-fat diet.

From balsamic to apple cider, there are numerous choices of vinegars available. When possible, shop for organic versions and avoid those that have added sugar for flavoring.

THE MEDITERRANEAN LIFESTYLE

Researchers concluded that it was not simply the diet in southern Greece and Crete which resulted in the healthiest population they examined. It was also how the Mediterranean populations lived that

Sunshine and Vitamin D

Spending time in the sun is vital to our health and well-being. Sunlight absorbed through the skin allows the body to produce Vitamin D. Although it's also available in certain foods such as fish and egg yolks, many people—regardless of diet—who are sedentary and spend a great deal of time indoors are often Vitamin D deficient which can result in a number of health problems including depression and a weakened immune system.

One thing that has not changed since the pre-1960s study of the Mediterranean lifestyle is the exposure to sun. Most modern residents of this area have ample blood levels of Vitamin D compared to other populations including Americans. Interestingly, if you are overweight you are likely to be low in Vitamin D because fat cells can extract it from the blood. Losing weight, getting out in the sun more (balancing your exposure with skin cancer risk), and consuming more dairy that is enriched in Vitamin D, such as the menu of the Slimmer program recommends, will help to remedy any deficiency and help you to feel healthier and happier.

had an enormous impact on their well-being, and it was clear that particular elements of the Mediterranean lifestyle were extremely relevant to their good health. Let's take a look at some of these important aspects and see how you can tap into them as you follow the Slimmer program.

Physical activity

Most participants of the Seven Countries Study in Greece lived in small rural towns where their livelihood was often based on some kind of physical activity. Farmers, olive pickers, builders, fishermen, and a number of other workers depended upon good physical fitness and strength in order to be able to do their jobs. As a result, simply by necessity, many of the participants were physically active and in remarkably good shape.

This isn't to say, however, that other residents were not physically active as well, although perhaps not as intensely. This is because, regardless of one's profession, a sedentary existence was not the norm. People walked everywhere, carried bundles and groceries with them, ran after children, danced, swam, helped neighbors with house projects and moving, and were generally up and about from the early morning until the late evening.

Today, most of us do not work in physically demanding professions. It is more likely that we sit behind a computer at our office or even at home, getting up only to grab another coffee or periodically stretch our legs. We get in the car to do our shopping and plop on the sofa in front of the TV after dinner, trying to relax after a stressful day. If we are lucky, we have a treadmill at home that we use or belong to a gym where we lift weights and exercise in the company of other stressed professionals.

Improving upon this scenario is actually a lot easier than it first appears. The answer lies in walking. Whenever we find ourselves needing to get from A to B, we should first think about getting there on our own two feet. Walking is probably the best exercise that any of us can immediately add to our lives. And there is a big difference between walking on a treadmill and walking outdoors through a park full of birds, flowers, and sunshine. Try it and see how rejuvenated you feel. If you can, aim to include a 20- to 30-minute outdoor pleasure walk each day, whether it be in the early morning, after lunch, or in the twilight hours. Also, make it a point to move as much as you can throughout the day. Choose low-impact but regular exercise such as walking up stairs instead of using the elevator.

My weight loss was helped by walking around, room to room, in my office and home after lunch! Find an easy way to incorporate a bit of exercise each day and you will feel the results.

Slower living

The Mediterranean lifestyle always conjures up visions of stress-free living, especially if you are vacationing there with the intention of getting away from it all. But is it really true that the year-round residents live a stress-free life too? Back in pre-1960s southern Greece it was certainly true, considering that high technology had yet to appear there. People were not rushing to catch commuter transport or navigating e-mails and cell phone calls every few minutes.

Today however, just about everywhere around the globe we are exposed to the stress that instant access to everything can create. Faster seems to be the buzzword and keeping up is not only encouraged but expected. Still, the Mediterranean, and to a great extent, the European approach to life has always contained an element of balance that many Americans have yet to learn. This isn't to say that you won't see Mediterraneans walking along the beach with a bluetooth in their ear or an iPad under their arms, but they somehow seem to know when it's time to disconnect and give their attention to the simpler things in life such as conversation, food, and fun. In fact, having an unhurried family meal in the middle of the day, followed by a brief nap and a rejuvenated afternoon return to work is still quite common. Although some Americans may not be able to follow this example, as healthy as it is, we can all certainly try to take quality time to relax and reconnect with the people in our lives that we love and the things in our lives that give us pleasure.

On a beautiful day, try to take a few moments at least to go outside, close your eyes, relax, and bask in the sun. Turn off your cell phone and turn on your iPod to listen to a favorite tune or a guided meditation. Finding moments when you can escape from the pressures of everyday living is an important part of creating a fulfilling and happy life, as well as contributing to your health and longevity.

Quality connections

Making quality time for our family and friends is only a part of how we can connect to the world around us. Many of the Study's Mediterranean participants also had a bond with nature, their environment, and their community. By spending more time outdoors it was natural that this would be the case. But connections like these run a bit deeper. There is a sense of history, ancestry, and belonging to the place where they live which can provide a healthy psychological and emotional balance to their existence. Many also had a spiritual connection, usually through their local church or place of worship. All of these elements, as simple as they seem, contribute to a population's appreciation of the natural progression of life—past, present, and future—and their place in it.

Years ago, before many families in America ended up with members on opposite coasts of the country from one another, there was a greater sense of a family's connection to community where, in many cases, generation after generation had been local citizens. Some of the more rural areas of America still retain a little of this history, but it is less and less common throughout the nation, particulary in suburban and urban areas. However, with the help of extended family additions, friends who are as close to you as relatives, and people who live nearby that you are kind and generous towards, you can create a solid sense of community of your own. Having this kind of connection can be one of the most rewarding and fulfilling aspects of modern life.

Volunteer to help at local facilities including libraries, senior centers, hospitals, and churches, and participate in other community activities and fund-raising events. Make time to chat with neighbors and patronize local businesses. Immerse yourself in your environment and become a part of it in the process.

Chapter 2

The Slimmer Program

LOVE AT FIRST TASTE

The Slimmer program has been specifically designed to maximize your weight loss in the healthiest way. Each day's menu contains important vitamins and minerals as well as ingredients that will help you to burn fat efficiently. This is why you should try to stick to each day's menu as closely as you can.

Similarly, each day's proportion of protein, fat, and carbohydrates has been carefully considered and should be followed as best you can. Based on my own research in dietetics here in Greece and recommendations from the World Health Organization as well as the USDA's MYPLATE program, these proportions have been confirmed to be most healthful. Extremes of any macronutrient—protein, fat, or carbs—are not generally recommended.

This doesn't mean, however, there is not any flexibility in the Slimmer program. If you come across a recipe that you don't care for, simply choose a menu from another day of the same cycle or the previous cycle. You can also make substitutions for equivalent foods listed in this chapter.

The Slimmer program is designed to be easy and stress-free, especially for working people. Read the Frequently Asked Questions for tips on saving time and effort on days when you are particularly busy and are unable to devote time to cooking or preparing meals.

Most important, the recipes you will be preparing will no doubt be some of the most delicious and flavorful you have ever enjoyed. Normally weight-loss diets can't make this type of claim, but Slimmer's recipes, many of which are based on traditional dishes served in my family's restaurant located in Fiscardo on the Greek island of Cefalonia, will surprise and delight you!

Maria and Eleni's Taverna

Fiscardo on Cefalonia island is one of the most beautiful and picturesque places in the world! It's blessed by God. Combining sea and mountain, the land is dotted with traditional eighteenth-century pastel-colored houses with tiled roofs and tiny balconies entwined with grapevines. By the sea are lovely traditional Greek tavernas (local restaurants) that overlook the crystal-blue water.

One of these tavernas belongs to my mum and her sister, Maria and Eleni. Everybody says: "Let's go to the two sisters' taverna to eat." In this taverna I spent all the summers of my life. I learned to love the fresh and natural flavors of the food, including those of homemade breads, crisp salads, fruity olive oil, and succulent fruit, and I was trained in the art of cooking by these two women, my mum and aunt, who I believe to be the best cooks in the world!

This knowledge of the art of cooking, along with my university studies in the science of dietology, contributed to my creation of the Slimmer health and diet program. In fact, after 2005 the family taverna menu was enriched with healthy, fat-burning and delicious Mediterranean dishes which were created by me and are of course included in the pages of this book.

Fiscardo attracts a great number of celebrities who arrive at its natural and quaint port on their luxurious yachts. Usually these celebrities visit Fiscardo in the late afternoon, go on a stroll in the lovely pebbled streets, and have lunch in the tavernas. Of course, they visit Maria and Eleni's Taverna, where they are warmly welcomed and served up some of the beloved recipes found in *Slimmer.* Steven Spielberg, Tom Hanks, and Rita Wilson are among the most frequent visitors, while Oprah Winfrey, Nicolas Cage, Penelope Cruz, Michelle Pfeiffer, Princess Diana, and Madonna have counted themselves as guests at the taverna as well. Because they are friendly, simple, ordinary people, we locals respect them and do not disturb them. That's why these celebrities visit us in Fiscardo again and again.

Madonna visited Maria and Eleni's Taverna in June 2000, when she was pregnant with her son Rocco. She ate the Slimmer Greek salad that my mother lovingly served with a big helping of traditional Greek rusk bread. She adored it. She asked for my mum at her table to meet her and then explained in tears that this dish reminded her of one of her mum's Italian meals that she used to prepare for her and her siblings: toasted bread topped with grated tomato, white cheese, olive oil, and basil.

The Cycles

Slimmer is divided into three separate Cycles—A, B, and C—consisting of 21 days each. Each day includes menu selections for breakfast, lunch, dinner, and even three healthy, light snacks—mid-morning, mid-afternoon, and bedtime. Although the three Cycles may at first glance appear quite similar, as they progress sequentially, each contains an increased amount of fat burning ingredients and combinations of foods that are vital to continued weight loss.

Although everyone is different, you can expect to lose about 10 percent of your weight in one month, and 5 percent of your weight each month after. Larger amounts of weight loss at the beginning are typical for many diets and most people will often slow down or even stop their rate of loss as they continue. This is why I have increased the amount of fat burning ingredients in Slimmer with each Cycle—it helps to counteract that trend.

Continue to go through the Cycles and repeat the program until you have reached your desired final Maintenance weight.

In addition to the menu selections, try to drink at least eight 8 oz glasses of water per day to assist your body in flushing out toxins and to keep you well hydrated. You can also have the following beverages:

- **Three cups of coffee per day**
- **Green or herbal tea each day**
- **Three diet sodas per week**

If you decide to switch or repeat a day's menu during the week, you should remember the following serving limitations:

- **Up to 3 servings of red meat in 1 week**
- **Up to 3 egg yolks in 1 week**
- **Up to 7 ounces of cheese in 1 week**

If you would like to select different fruits than the ones specified in any menu or recipe, use the following fruit equivalents when making substitutions:

APPLE, ONE MEDIUM =

APRICOTS, FRESH, TWO MEDIUM =

BANANA, HALF A MEDIUM FRUIT =

CACTUS PEAR, ONE MEDIUM =

CHERRIES, ONE CUP =

DATES, TWO MEDIUM =

FIGS, FRESH, ONE MEDIUM =

GRAPES, ONE CUP =

GRAPEFRUIT, HALF A LARGE FRUIT =

GRAPEFRUIT JUICE, HALF A GLASS =

KIWI FRUIT, TWO MEDIUM =

MELON, ONE MEDIUM SLICE =

BLACKBERRIES, ONE CUP =

BLUEBERRIES, HALF A CUP =

ORANGE, ONE MEDIUM =

ORANGE JUICE, HALF A GLASS =

PEACH OR NECTARINE, ONE MEDIUM =

PEAR, ONE MEDIUM =

PLUMS, TWO MEDIUM =

POMEGRANATE, ONE MEDIUM =

PRUNES, THREE MEDIUM =

STRAWBERRIES, ONE CUP =

TANGERINES OR CLEMENTINES, TWO SMALL =

WATERMELON, A THIN SLICE.

And if you feel like having something in between your meals and snacks, you may munch on 3 plain cucumber or carrot sticks.

Slimmer Burns Fat Like No Other Diet

Slimmer incorporates recent dietary findings about specific foods and their combinations that help you to burn fat. Here are some of the highlights you will find in the Slimmer program:

- **Low-fat dairy increases your metabolism (Slimmer recommends milk, yogurt, and/or cheese consumption every day).**
- **Spicy mustard (in dressings and sauces) can increase your metabolism by up to 25 percent for several hours after ingestion (spicy food causes a**

spike in internal temperatures, causing the body to burn more calories).

- Fiber-rich oats and whole grains (eaten at breakfast and in the recipes) help to increase fat burning.
- Lean protein (eaten often on the Slimmer program) increases metabolism while lean beef and eggs help burn belly fat due to this increase.
- Salmon and tuna (eaten often on the Slimmer program) reduce leptin levels and increase metabolism.
- Protein-rich plant sources such as beans, pulses, and brown rice (eaten often on the Slimmer program) can increase metabolism and fat burning by 30 percent.
- Salads dressed with lemon or vinegar (eaten every day) provide ultimate fat burning.
- In addition, each day's breakfast should contain a high-fiber, antioxidant- and vitamin-rich fruit, as well as your choice of coffee or tea.

The Power of Life Blend

To ensure you are getting the utmost nutrition and fiber on a daily basis, and to add interest and flavor to your dishes, Slimmer's Power of Life Blend is a mixture you will want to create on a regular basis and have on hand to sprinkle onto cereal, soups and salads, entrees, and fruit and yogurt. This blend's nutritional content—in the form of plant protein, fiber, healthy omega-3 fatty acids, and important minerals such as calcium and potassium—will keep you satiated and energized.

Simply combine the following ingredients in a blender or processor and pulverize until powder-like:

- **1 cup hulled sunflower seeds**
- **1 cup hulled pumpkin seeds**
- **1 cup flax seeds**
- **1 cup sesame seeds**

Use up to 2 teaspoons per day and store in the refrigerator for freshness.

Free Days

Slimmer rewards you for your dedication and adherence to the program by allowing for Free Days. On these occasions you can actually enjoy a favorite food at lunch or dinner that is not normally considered a diet choice. For example, you might want to have a cheeseburger or a serving of fried chicken. Maybe baby back ribs would be your choice, or veal parmesan.

Whatever you select you must remember one rule. Instead of fries with your cheeseburger or a buttermilk biscuit with your fried chicken, always have a salad as your accompaniment. Similarly, shun the mashed potatoes or side of spaghetti and opt for the salad. The rest of your meals on that day can be any that you choose from that Cycle. And best of all, you may enjoy two Happy Moments on Free Days!

REWARD YOURSELF
ENJOY YOUR "HAPPY MOMENT"

So, what exactly are Happy Moments and how do they fit into the Slimmer program?

If there is something that you particularly like which is not a part of the diet (such as chocolate!) you can enjoy a small indulgence every day as a flavorful Happy Moment. For example, you might enjoy a low-fat cereal bar during the afternoon or a small scoop of ice cream after dinner. These can be included as Happy Moments and you will find that they will help tremendously in sticking to the Slimmer program. Having a Happy Moment to look forward to can mean all the difference between giving up in a weak moment and finding the motivation to carry on with your weight-loss journey.

Some people like to enjoy their Happy Moments at the same time with the same treat every day. For example, a low-fat cappuccino after lunch, or a small chocolate chip cookie in the afternoon. It is really up to you how you plan your Happy Moment each day. And remember that on Free Days you can enjoy two Happy Moments!

Here are some ideas for including flavorful Happy Moments in your daily Slimmer menu:

- **Regular coffee (with half and half) and a teaspoon of raw sugar**
- **Cappuccino with a teaspoon of raw sugar**
- **Low-fat hot chocolate**
- **1 cup reduced fat chocolate, strawberry, or vanilla milk**
- **Small reduced fat pudding**
- **Small serving Jell-O**

- 1 scoop reduced fat ice cream, frozen yogurt, or sorbet
- 1 ounce dark chocolate
- 1 medium cookie
- 4 oz dry white or red wine
- 6 oz light beer
- 1 small alcoholic drink
- 9 plain almonds or walnuts
- 1 100-calorie snack pack of your choice

Here are some quick Happy Moment recipe ideas you could also enjoy:

Orange Fizz

Mix half a glass of club soda with half a glass of fresh orange juice and a teaspoon of natural, unprocessed sugar (optional). Add ice and serve.

Red Fruit Smoothie

In a blender, puree 1 cup of your choice of red fruit (such as strawberries, raspberries etc.) with 3 tablespoons of low-fat yogurt of the same flavor and 3 tablespoons of low-fat milk.

How to Enjoy Your Flavorful Happy Moment

Place a slice of Slimmer Apple Pie on a pretty plate, and place it on the table. Sit and try to relax, knowing that you deserve this moment of pleasure. Look at the apple pie for a while and then cut it up into smaller pieces. Notice what the pieces look like: the golden, crispy pastry, the grated apple, the round, white bits of cottage cheese, the small, dark raisins, and the manner in which they all blend harmoniously.

Take a piece of the apple pie, bring it close to your nose, and smell the wonderful aroma, the result of all the ingredients and especially the sensual, bittersweet scent of the cinnamon. Now, close your eyes and take your first bite. Chew well, enjoying the flavor. Continue to eat your pie in the same manner. Don't forget to express your gratitude for this flavorful experience.

You must enjoy all your meals in the slow, conscious manner that you enjoyed your Slimmer Apple Pie. Don't forget that the most important thing is to enjoy every moment of your meal, as if you were eating that particular food for the first time, with no trace of daily anxiety and stress. This is the traditional Mediterranean approach to food and one which is worth bringing back to the modern table.

If you follow the above advice faithfully, it is certain that you will discover the greatness of sensual stimulation while eating, which you must then apply to the rest of your life. Let yourself feel the incredible smoothness of a small piece of chocolate as it melts in your mouth, observe the colors of a flower and enjoy its aroma, walk on a beach and listen to the waves . . .

All of these are sensual experiences that you can bring on by concentrating, and with practice. In this way, you can learn to appreciate the "small" things, the "small" pleasures in life. Beginning to enjoy every moment of your life will become your best defense against the destructive emotions you may sometimes feel because of mistakes or failures that you will undoubtedly face at some time in your life. If you learn to enjoy, you won't seek a solution in consuming unhealthy food, desserts, or alcohol.

Fruity Italian Ice

In a blender, puree the following: 1 cut-up ripe fruit (such as a peach, part of pineapple, or banana), a teaspoon of natural, unprocessed sugar (optional), a few drops of lemon juice, some lemon zest, 1/4 cup crushed ice, and a cup of cold water. Process until smooth.

Strawberry or Banana Ice Cream

Slice a cup of strawberries or a small banana (drizzled with lemon juice) and freeze. Add to a blender along with 1/2 cup of very cold condensed milk (4% fat) and a tablespoon of natural, unprocessed sugar. Process until creamy and smooth.

Strawberries with Brandy Banana Cream

Wash and hull 1 cup of strawberries and place in a serving dish. Make a cream to pour on top by blending together 1 teaspoon brandy, 2 tablespoons low-fat Greek yogurt, and half a small, ripe banana. Finally, sprinkle with a teaspoon of brown sugar.

Banana Pudding with Cinnamon

In a blender combine 3 tablespoons of low-fat Greek yogurt, half a medium ripe banana, and a teaspoon of honey. Pour into a bowl and sprinkle with a little ground cinnamon.

Chocolate Banana

Drizzle a small, ripe banana with a few drops of lemon juice, and wrap in foil. Place in the freezer for 2 hours. Melt together 1 tablespoon of low-fat milk and a small piece of dark chocolate in a small pot or in the microwave. Leaving the banana in the foil, use a pastry brush to coat the banana with the chocolate. Refrigerate for 1 hour, slice, and serve.

Pineapple with Chocolate Sauce

Place 2 fresh pineapple rings in a small serving bowl. Melt together 1 tablespoon of low-fat milk and a small piece of dark chocolate in a small pot or in the microwave. Pour over the pineapple and serve.

Chocolate Dipped Orange

Wash a small orange, cut away some of the rind (leaving a few strips), and cut into thin slices. Put the slices in a pot with 1/3 cup of water and 1 tablespoon of natural, unprocessed sugar. Simmer over low heat until the slices are soft, about 20 minutes. Drain the slices well and place on waxed or parchment paper. Melt together 1 tablespoon of low-fat milk and a small piece of dark chocolate in a small pot or in the microwave. Dip half of each orange slice into the chocolate, lay on the paper, and allow to cool before serving.

Chocolate Almond Prunes

Soak 3 prunes in brandied water or iced tea overnight in the refrigerator. Drain, pat dry, and stuff each prune with an unsalted, blanched almond (or half a walnut). Melt together 1 tablespoon of low-fat milk and a small piece of dark chocolate in a small pot or in the microwave. Dip each stuffed prune in the chocolate, lay on the paper, and allow to cool before serving.

Jell-O with Yogurt

Dissolve a package of light fruit Jell-O in 1 cup of hot water and stir well until it has dissolved. Pour into a large bowl, add a cup of cold water and stir. Allow to cool for 10 minutes, then stir in 1 cup of low-fat Greek yogurt and blend well. Pour into three small dessert dishes and refrigerate until firm, stirring occasionally.

Slimmer Baked Apple

Peel and core an apple and cut into 1/4-inch rounds. Place the slices in a nonstick, ovenproof dish and bake at 350° F for about 10 minutes, until they are golden brown. Turn the slices over. Mix a teaspoon of natural, unprocessed sugar and a teaspoon of cinnamon

Creating Happy Moments in Your Mind

Not all Happy Moments have to be about food and treats. Did you know that the same brain chemical—dopamine—that make us feel so good eating chocolate is also released when we are simply gleeful and joyful? Laughter can flood our brains with such pleasure that some people often feel "high" after a good giggle. The same can be true after a relaxing daydream.

Try to create as many of these types of Happy Moments as you can throughout your day. Close your eyes and think of a funny incident that made you laugh. Or imagine that you are walking along the beach of a secluded Greek island and can feel the warm sand between your toes and the salty sea breeze on your face. When you sip your red wine, imagine you are in the Mediterranean in a vineyard fragrant with grapes and glowing with sunshine. These types of meditations, often referred to as mindfulness, can be enormously stress relieving and healthy for your body, mind, and spirit. Try to elicit the exact "happy" emotion associated with the imagery, and notice how good you suddenly feel.

together and sprinkle over the apple slices. Bake for 2 more minutes. Serve warm or at room temperature.

Slimmer Apple Pie

Peel, core, and grate 2 medium apples. Mix together with 1 cup well-drained, low-fat small curd cottage cheese, 2 tablespoons of raisins, and a dash of ground cinnamon. Lay 2 phyllo pastry sheets in a small nonstick, ovenproof dish. Spoon the filling onto one side of the pastry and then roll it over to make a strudel shape. Brush a teaspoon of melted butter on the pastry and bake at 350° F for about 15 minutes, until golden. Makes 2 servings.

Getting Ready

Before you actually begin Cycle A of the Slimmer program, getting yourself ready, mentally and emotionally, is a good idea. Think about the following, which will help you prepare for your weight-loss journey:

Assess your present dietary habits, the state of your health, and your lifestyle in general. Start a food diary today, and note down everything you eat for a week. Jot down not only the kind of food and the quantity, but also where you eat and when you eat.

As soon as you finish the diary, study it well and note if anything jumps out at you. Are there foods that you consume in large quantities (such as chocolate, cookies, potato chips, soft drinks)? Ask yourself if you can completely avoid some of these treats without even noticing. If your answer is yes, begin to do so now. Don't wait for the diet to begin. If complete elimination is too much, gradually reduce the amount you consume of this particular food. Begin to transform uncontrolled eating into healthy, controlled eating.

Reinvent Yourself

At this early stage of thinking you can already begin to redefine your dietary habits. Choose just one small change that you think will be easy for you to achieve. For example, make a decision to drink more water during the day, rather than carbonated soft drinks that contain sugar or sugar substitutes. Then put your decision into action and remember that if you do not succeed immediately you should never give up. Try again and again. Believe it or not, "failure" is one of the most important things you can learn from when creating new diet habits and you will find all of these experiences useful when you officially start the Slimmer program. You can understand a lot about yourself if you carefully examine exactly what it was that kept you from your goal and be better prepared the next time.

You should also get physically ready to begin. How? When you decide to start the Slimmer program, it must become your number-one priority. Prepare for it. Get plenty of good quality sleep in the days and even weeks before, so you are rested and feeling as vital as you can. Remove as much stress from your life as you can. Begin meditating or doing yoga or a walking routine each day. Having too many issues at once to worry about and not feeling physically able to handle a new challenge will exhaust your energies and make it more difficult for you to succeed.

Now is your time! So be good to yourself and know that what you are about to begin will change your life forever.

Your Greek Island Vacation

Since so much of the Slimmer program you are about to enjoy is based on the healthy eating and living of the wonderful Mediterranean, why not imagine that you are embarking on a Greek island vacation?

Sound impossible? Here's how:

As you begin your morning with a bite of fresh fruit, imagine that you have picked it yourself from the plentiful fruit trees outside your window. Taste the sunshine in its natural sweetness and savor the flavor.

When you take a spoonful of rich and creamy Greek yogurt, imagine basking in the sun with the warm breeze of the Mediterranean Sea gently touching your skin.

Hear the soft sounds of the coastal waters as you sip a bit of wine and enjoy your dinner of freshly grilled fish and tender salad greens on the porch of your beach cottage.

Gaze up at the stars as you slowly sip a cup of warm, fresh milk to lull you into a night of peaceful sleep.

And perhaps best of all, imagine how great it feels being healthy and slim when you embark on your real Greek island vacation as a reward for a job well done on the Slimmer program!

The Slimmer Cycles

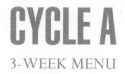

CYCLE A
3-WEEK MENU

DAY 1

BREAKFAST:

1 large orange, 2 medium kiwi, or 3 bite-size prunes

1/4 cup whole grain or bran cereal

3/4 cup reduced fat (1%) milk

1 slice whole wheat / whole grain bread, toasted (if desired) with

1 oz reduced fat cheese (see FAQs)

Coffee or tea (green or herbal)

MID-MORNING SNACK:

Low-fat fruit-flavored yogurt (6 oz)

LUNCH:

Slimmer Chef's Salad (page 105)

2 thin breadsticks or rye crackers

MID-AFTERNOON SNACK:

Cinnamon Apple Greek Yogurt (page 134)

DINNER:

Slimmer Chicken à la Crème (page 117)

Large tossed salad (see FAQs)

BEDTIME SNACK:

6 oz reduced fat (1%) milk or plain yogurt

DAY 2

BREAKFAST:

1 large orange, 2 medium kiwi, or 3 bite-size prunes

1/4 cup whole grain or bran cereal

3/4 cup reduced fat (1%) milk

1 slice whole wheat / whole grain bread, toasted (if desired) with

2 tsp fruit jam or honey

Coffee or tea (green or herbal)

MID-MORNING SNACK:

Low-fat fruit-flavored yogurt (6 oz)

LUNCH:

Slimmer Chicken à la Crème (from Day 1 dinner; page 117)

Large tossed salad

MID-AFTERNOON SNACK:

Two fruit selections of choice

DINNER:

Spaghetti Bolognese (page 120)

Large tossed salad

BEDTIME SNACK:

6 oz reduced fat (1%) milk or yogurt

DAY 3

BREAKFAST:

1 large orange, 2 medium kiwi, or 3 bite-size prunes

1/4 cup whole grain or bran cereal

3/4 cup reduced fat (1%) milk

1 slice whole wheat / whole grain bread, toasted (if desired) with

1 boiled or poached egg

Coffee or tea (green or herbal)

MID-MORNING SNACK:

Low-fat fruit-flavored yogurt (6 oz)

LUNCH:

Slimmer Greek Salad (page 106)

2 thin breadsticks or rye crackers

MID-AFTERNOON SNACK:

Two fruit selections of choice

DINNER:

Mediterranean Burger (page 121)

Large tossed salad

BEDTIME SNACK:

6 oz reduced fat (1%) milk or yogurt

DAY 4

BREAKFAST:

1 large orange, 2 medium kiwi, or 3 bite-size prunes

1/4 cup whole grain or bran cereal

3/4 cup reduced fat (1%) milk

1 slice whole wheat / whole grain bread, toasted (if desired)
with 1 oz reduced fat cheese

Coffee or tea (green or herbal)

MID-MORNING SNACK:

Low-fat fruit-flavored yogurt (6 oz)

_____

LUNCH:

Tomato and Lentil Soup (page 111)

Large tossed salad

MID-AFTERNOON SNACK:

1 cup red fruit (choose from cherries, red grapes, or strawberries)

_____

DINNER:

Pepperoni Pita Pizza (page 113)

Large tossed salad

BEDTIME SNACK:

6 oz reduced fat (1%) milk or yogurt

DAY 5

BREAKFAST:

1 large orange, 2 medium kiwi, or 3 bite-size prunes

1/4 cup whole grain or bran cereal

3/4 cup reduced fat (1%) milk

1 slice whole wheat / whole grain bread, toasted (if desired) with

2 slices turkey bacon

Coffee or tea (green or herbal)

MID-MORNING SNACK:

Low-fat fruit-flavored yogurt (6 oz)

LUNCH:

Pasta Salad Primavera (page 110)

MID-AFTERNOON SNACK:

2 fruit selections of choice

DINNER:

Sole with Oregano and Lemon (page 125)

Large tossed salad

BEDTIME SNACK:

6 oz reduced fat (1%) milk or yogurt

DAY 6

BREAKFAST:

1 large orange, 2 medium kiwi, or 3 bite-size prunes

1/4 cup whole grain or bran cereal

3/4 cup reduced fat (1%) milk

1 slice whole wheat / whole grain bread, toasted (if desired) with

2 small turkey sausages

Coffee or tea (green or herbal)

MID-MORNING SNACK:

Low-fat fruit-flavored yogurt (6 oz)

LUNCH:

Slimmer Chef's Salad (page 105)

MID-AFTERNOON SNACK:

1 cup red fruit (choose from cherries, red grapes, or strawberries)

DINNER:

Easy Seafood Risotto (page 128)

Large tossed salad

BEDTIME SNACK:

6 oz reduced fat (1%) milk or yogurt

DAY 7

Choose any day's menu from Cycle A or have a FREE DAY! (See page 29 to read all about Free Days.)

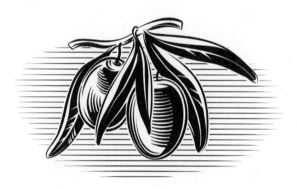

DAY 8

BREAKFAST:

1 large orange, 2 medium kiwi, or 3 bite-size prunes

1/4 cup whole grain or bran cereal

3/4 cup reduced fat (1%) milk

1 slice whole wheat / whole grain bread, toasted (if desired) with

1 oz reduced fat cheese

Coffee or tea (green or herbal)

MID-MORNING SNACK:

Low-fat fruit-flavored yogurt (6 oz)

LUNCH:

Easy Seafood Risotto (from Day 6 dinner; page 128)

Large tossed salad

MID-AFTERNOON SNACK:

2 fruit selections of choice

DINNER:

Greek Chicken with Roast Potatoes (page 118)

Large tossed salad

BEDTIME SNACK:

6 oz reduced fat (1%) milk or yogurt

DAY 9

BREAKFAST:

1 large orange, 2 medium kiwi, or 3 bite-size prunes

1/4 cup whole grain or bran cereal

3/4 cup reduced fat (1%) milk

1 slice whole wheat / whole grain bread, toasted (if desired) with

2 tsp fruit jam or honey

Coffee or tea (green or herbal)

MID-MORNING SNACK:

Low-fat fruit-flavored yogurt (6 oz)

LUNCH:

Greek Chicken with Roast Potatoes (from Day 8 dinner; page 118)

Large tossed salad

MID-AFTERNOON SNACK:

2 fruit selections of choice

DINNER:

Veal or Pork Provençal (page 124)

Large tossed salad

BEDTIME SNACK:

6 oz reduced fat (1%) milk or yogurt

DAY 10

BREAKFAST:

1 large orange, 2 medium kiwi, or 3 bite-size prunes

1/4 cup whole grain or bran cereal

3/4 cup reduced fat (1%) milk

1 slice whole wheat / whole grain bread, toasted (if desired) with

2 slices turkey bacon

Coffee or tea (green or herbal)

MID-MORNING SNACK:

Low-fat fruit-flavored yogurt (6 oz)

LUNCH:

Three Bean Soup (page 112)

Large tossed salad

MID-AFTERNOON SNACK:

1 cup red fruit (choose from cherries, red grapes, or strawberries)

DINNER:

Slimmer Greek Salad Pizza (page 115)

Large tossed salad

BEDTIME SNACK:

6 oz reduced fat (1%) milk or yogurt

DAY 11

BREAKFAST:

1 large orange, 2 medium kiwi, or 3 bite-size prunes

1/4 cup whole grain or bran cereal

3/4 cup reduced fat (1%) milk

1 slice whole wheat / whole grain bread, toasted (if desired) with

1 boiled or poached egg

Coffee or tea (green or herbal)

MID-MORNING SNACK:

Low-fat fruit-flavored yogurt (6 oz)

LUNCH:

Slimmer Greek Salad (page 106)

2 thin breadsticks or rye crackers

MID-AFTERNOON SNACK:

Fruit Salad with Yogurt Crunch (page 133)

DINNER:

Beefsteak Florentine (page 123)

Large tossed salad

BEDTIME SNACK:

6 oz reduced fat (1%) milk or yogurt

DAY 12

BREAKFAST:

1 large orange, 2 medium kiwi, or 3 bite-size prunes

1/4 cup whole grain or bran cereal

3/4 cup reduced fat (1%) milk

1 slice whole wheat / whole grain bread, toasted (if desired) with

2 small turkey sausages

Coffee or tea (green or herbal)

MID-MORNING SNACK:

Low-fat fruit-flavored yogurt (6 oz)

_____

LUNCH:

Salmon Salad with Honey and Balsamic Dressing (page 107)

MID-AFTERNOON SNACK:

1 cup red fruit (choose from cherries, red grapes, or strawberries)

_____

DINNER:

Mediterranean Mac and Cheese (page 129)

Large tossed salad

BEDTIME SNACK:

6 oz reduced fat (1%) milk or yogurt

DAY 13

BREAKFAST:

1 large orange, 2 medium kiwi, or 3 bite-size prunes

1/4 cup whole grain or bran cereal

3/4 cup reduced fat (1%) milk

1 slice whole wheat / whole grain bread, toasted (if desired) with

2 slices turkey bacon

Coffee or tea (green or herbal)

MID-MORNING SNACK:

Low-fat fruit-flavored yogurt (6 oz)

——————

LUNCH:

Slimmer Chef's Salad (page 105)

2 thin breadsticks or rye crackers

MID-AFTERNOON SNACK:

Banana Walnut Yogurt (page 135)

——————

DINNER:

Baked Fish and Vegetables Aegean Style (page 126)

Large tossed salad

BEDTIME SNACK:

6 oz reduced fat (1%) milk or yogurt

DAY 14

Choose any day's menu from Cycle A or have a FREE DAY! (See page 29 to read all about Free Days.)

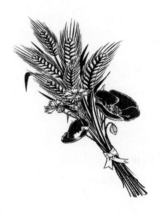

DAY 15

BREAKFAST:

1 large orange, 2 medium kiwi, or 3 bite-size prunes

1/4 cup whole grain or bran cereal

3/4 cup reduced fat (1%) milk

1 slice whole wheat / whole grain bread, toasted (if desired) with

1 oz reduced fat cheese

Coffee or tea (green or herbal)

MID-MORNING SNACK:

Low-fat fruit-flavored yogurt (6 oz)

LUNCH:

Pasta Salad Primavera (page 110)

MID-AFTERNOON SNACK:

2 fruit selections of choice

DINNER:

Greek-style Sliders with Yogurt Sauce (page 122)

Large tossed salad

BEDTIME SNACK:

6 oz reduced fat (1%) milk or yogurt

DAY 16

BREAKFAST:

1 large orange, 2 medium kiwi, or 3 bite-size prunes

1/4 cup whole grain or bran cereal

3/4 cup reduced fat (1%) milk

1 slice whole wheat / whole grain bread, toasted (if desired) with

3 Tablespoons low-fat cottage cheese

Coffee or tea (green or herbal)

MID-MORNING SNACK:

Low-fat fruit-flavored yogurt (6 oz)

LUNCH:

Greek-style Sliders with Yogurt Sauce (from Day 15 dinner; page 122)

Large tossed salad

MID-AFTERNOON SNACK:

2 fruit selections of choice

DINNER:

Chicken Stew with Garden Peas (page 119)

Large tossed salad

BEDTIME SNACK:

6 oz reduced fat (1%) milk or yogurt

DAY 17

BREAKFAST:

1 large orange, 2 medium kiwi, or 3 bite-size prunes

1/4 cup whole grain or bran cereal

3/4 cup reduced fat (1%) milk

1 slice whole wheat / whole grain bread, toasted (if desired) with

2 slices turkey bacon

Coffee or tea (green or herbal)

MID-MORNING SNACK:

Low-fat fruit-flavored yogurt (6 oz)

LUNCH:

Chicken Stew with Garden Peas (from Day 16 dinner; page 119)

Large tossed salad

MID-AFTERNOON SNACK:

Slimmer Fruit Salad (page 132)

DINNER:

Pasta Puttanesca (page 130)

Large tossed salad

BEDTIME SNACK:

6 oz reduced fat (1%) milk or yogurt

DAY 18

BREAKFAST:

1 large orange, 2 medium kiwi, or 3 bite-size prunes

1/4 cup whole grain or bran cereal

3/4 cup reduced fat (1%) milk

1 slice whole wheat / whole grain bread, toasted (if desired) with

2 small turkey sausages

Coffee or tea (green or herbal)

MID-MORNING SNACK:

Low-fat fruit-flavored yogurt (6 oz)

LUNCH:

Slimmer Egg Salad Pita (page 109)

Large tossed salad

MID-AFTERNOON SNACK:

Pear and Yogurt Parfait (page 136)

DINNER:

Shrimp with Lemon Sauce (page 127)

Large tossed salad

BEDTIME SNACK:

6 oz reduced fat (1%) milk or yogurt

DAY 19

It's a Free Day!

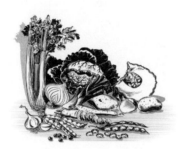

DAY 20

BREAKFAST:

1 large orange, 2 medium kiwi, or 3 bite-size prunes

1/4 cup whole grain or bran cereal

3/4 cup reduced fat (1%) milk

1 slice whole wheat / whole grain bread, toasted (if desired) with

2 tsp fruit jam or honey

Coffee or tea (green or herbal)

MID-MORNING SNACK:

Low-fat fruit-flavored yogurt (6 oz)

LUNCH:

Mediterranean Tuna Salad (page 108)

1/2 medium whole wheat pita

MID-AFTERNOON SNACK:

Cinnamon Apple Greek Yogurt (page 134)

DINNER:

Slimmer Loaded Baked Potato (page 131)

Large tossed salad

BEDTIME SNACK:

6 oz reduced fat (1%) milk or yogurt

DAY 21

Choose any day's menu from Cycle A or have a FREE DAY! (See page 29 to read all about Free Days.)

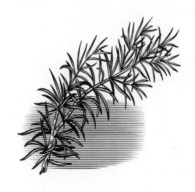

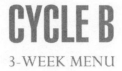

CYCLE B
3-WEEK MENU

DAY 1

BREAKFAST:

1 large orange, 2 medium kiwi, or 3 bite-size prunes

1/4 cup whole grain or bran cereal

3/4 cup reduced fat (1%) milk

1 slice whole wheat / whole grain bread, toasted (if desired) with

1 oz reduced fat cheese

Coffee or tea (green or herbal)

MID-MORNING SNACK:

Low-fat fruit-flavored yogurt (6 oz)

LUNCH:

Slimmer Shrimp Salad (page 139)

MID-AFTERNOON SNACK:

Fruit salad with yogurt (see FAQs)

DINNER:

Chicken with Orzo (page 151)

Large tossed salad

BEDTIME SNACK:

6 oz reduced fat (1%) milk or plain yogurt

DAY 2

BREAKFAST:

1 large orange, 2 medium kiwi, or 3 bite-size prunes

1/4 cup whole grain or bran cereal

3/4 cup reduced fat (1%) milk

1 slice whole wheat / whole grain bread, toasted (if desired) with

2 tsp fruit jam or honey

Coffee or tea (green or herbal)

MID-MORNING SNACK:

Low-fat fruit-flavored yogurt (6 oz)

LUNCH:

Chicken with Orzo (from Day 1 dinner; page 151)

Large tossed salad

MID-AFTERNOON SNACK:

Two fruit selections of choice

DINNER:

Slimmer Baked Ziti (page 162)

Large tossed salad

BEDTIME SNACK:

6 oz reduced fat (1%) milk or yogurt

DAY 3

BREAKFAST:

1 large orange, 2 medium kiwi, or 3 bite-size prunes

1/4 cup whole grain or bran cereal

3/4 cup reduced fat (1%) milk

1 slice whole wheat / whole grain bread, toasted (if desired) with

1 boiled or poached egg

Coffee or tea (green or herbal)

MID-MORNING SNACK:

Low-fat fruit-flavored yogurt (6 oz)

LUNCH:

White Bean Soup (page 147)

Large tossed salad

MID-AFTERNOON SNACK:

Fruit salad with yogurt

DINNER:

Greek-style Meatballs with Rice (page 156)

Large tossed salad

BEDTIME SNACK:

6 oz reduced fat (1%) milk or yogurt

DAY 4

BREAKFAST:

1 large orange, 2 medium kiwi, or 3 bite-size prunes

1/4 cup whole grain or bran cereal

3/4 cup reduced fat (1%) milk

1 slice whole wheat / whole grain bread, toasted (if desired) with

1 oz reduced fat cheese

Coffee or tea (green or herbal)

MID-MORNING SNACK:

Low-fat fruit-flavored yogurt (6 oz)

LUNCH:

Greek-style Meatballs with Rice (from Day 3 dinner; page 156)

Large tossed salad

MID-AFTERNOON SNACK:

1 cup red fruit (choose from cherries, red grapes, or strawberries)

DINNER:

Slimmer Sausage Pizza (page 148)

Large tossed salad

BEDTIME SNACK:

6 oz reduced fat (1%) milk or yogurt

DAY 5

BREAKFAST:

1 large orange, 2 medium kiwi, or 3 bite-size prunes

1/4 cup whole grain or bran cereal

3/4 cup reduced fat (1%) milk

1 slice whole wheat / whole grain bread, toasted (if desired) with

2 slices turkey bacon

Coffee or tea (green or herbal)

MID-MORNING SNACK:

Low-fat fruit-flavored yogurt (6 oz)

LUNCH:

Slimmer Potato and Egg Salad (page 140)

MID-AFTERNOON SNACK:

Orange Banana Chocolate Crisp (page 164)

DINNER:

Citrus Glazed Salmon (page 159)

3/4 cup brown rice

Large tossed salad

BEDTIME SNACK:

6 oz reduced fat (1%) milk or yogurt

DAY 6

BREAKFAST:

1 large orange, 2 medium kiwi, or 3 bite-size prunes

1/4 cup whole grain or bran cereal

3/4 cup reduced fat (1%) milk

1 slice whole wheat / whole grain bread, toasted (if desired) with

2 small turkey sausages

Coffee or tea (green or herbal)

MID-MORNING SNACK:

Low-fat fruit-flavored yogurt (6 oz)

LUNCH:

Citrus Glazed Salmon (from Day 5 dinner; page 159)

3/4 cup brown rice

Large tossed salad

MID-AFTERNOON SNACK:

1 cup red fruit (choose from cherries, red grapes, or strawberries)

DINNER:

Garden Vegetable Omelette (page 150)

Large tossed salad

BEDTIME SNACK:

6 oz reduced fat (1%) milk or yogurt

DAY 7

Choose any day's menu from Cycle A or B or have a FREE DAY!

(See page 29 to read all about Free Days.)

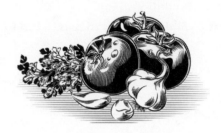

DAY 8

BREAKFAST:

1 large orange, 2 medium kiwi, or 3 bite-size prunes

1/4 cup whole grain or bran cereal

3/4 cup reduced fat (1%) milk

1 slice whole wheat / whole grain bread, toasted (if desired) with

1 oz reduced fat cheese

Coffee or tea (green or herbal)

MID-MORNING SNACK:

Low-fat fruit-flavored yogurt (6 oz)

LUNCH:

Salmon Salad Platter (page 141)

1/2 medium whole wheat pita

MID-AFTERNOON SNACK:

Fruit salad with yogurt

DINNER:

Herb Roasted Chicken with Vegetables (page 152)

Large tossed salad

BEDTIME SNACK:

6 oz reduced fat (1%) milk or yogurt

DAY 9

BREAKFAST:

1 large orange, 2 medium kiwi, or 3 bite-size prunes

1/4 cup whole grain or bran cereal

3/4 cup reduced fat (1%) milk

1 slice whole wheat / whole grain bread, toasted (if desired) with

2 tsp fruit jam or honey

Coffee or tea (green or herbal)

MID-MORNING SNACK:

Low-fat fruit-flavored yogurt (6 oz)

LUNCH:

Herb Roasted Chicken with Vegetables (from Day 8 dinner; page 152)

Small whole grain roll

Large tossed salad

MID-AFTERNOON SNACK:

2 fruit selections of choice

DINNER:

Skillet Steak with Mushrooms (page 157)

Large tossed salad

BEDTIME SNACK:

6 oz reduced fat (1%) milk or yogurt

DAY 10

BREAKFAST:

1 large orange, 2 medium kiwi, or 3 bite-size prunes

1/4 cup whole grain or bran cereal

3/4 cup reduced fat (1%) milk

1 slice whole wheat / whole grain bread, toasted (if desired) with

2 slices turkey bacon

Coffee or tea (green or herbal)

MID-MORNING SNACK:

Low-fat fruit-flavored yogurt (6 oz)

LUNCH:

Bean and Vegetable Chowder (page 146)

Large tossed salad

MID-AFTERNOON SNACK:

1 cup red fruit (choose from cherries, red grapes, or strawberries)

DINNER:

Slimmer Linguine with Shrimp (page 161)

Large tossed salad

BEDTIME SNACK:

6 oz reduced fat (1%) milk or yogurt

DAY 11

It's a Free Day!

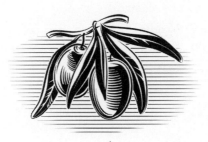

DAY 12

BREAKFAST:

1 large orange, 2 medium kiwi, or 3 bite-size prunes

1/4 cup whole grain or bran cereal

3/4 cup reduced fat (1%) milk

1 slice whole wheat / whole grain bread, toasted (if desired) with

2 small turkey sausages

Coffee or tea (green or herbal)

MID-MORNING SNACK:

Low-fat fruit-flavored yogurt (6 oz)

LUNCH:

Slimmer Club Sandwich (page 145)

Large tossed salad

MID-AFTERNOON SNACK:

1 cup red fruit (choose from cherries, red grapes, or strawberries)

DINNER:

Greek-style Phyllo Calzone (page 149)

Large tossed salad

BEDTIME SNACK:

6 oz reduced fat (1%) milk or yogurt

DAY 13

BREAKFAST:

1 large orange, 2 medium kiwi, or 3 bite-size prunes

1/4 cup whole grain or bran cereal

3/4 cup reduced fat (1%) milk

1 slice whole wheat / whole grain bread, toasted (if desired) with

2 slices turkey bacon

Coffee or tea (green or herbal)

MID-MORNING SNACK:

Low-fat fruit-flavored yogurt (6 oz)

LUNCH:

Greek-style Phyllo Calzone (from Day 12 dinner; page 149)

Large tossed salad

MID-AFTERNOON SNACK:

Fruit salad with yogurt

DINNER:

Spicy Sautéed Veal Chop (page 158)

Large tossed salad

BEDTIME SNACK:

6 oz reduced fat (1%) milk or yogurt

DAY 14

Choose any day's menu from Cycle A or B or have a FREE DAY! (See page 29 to read all about Free Days.)

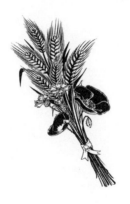

DAY 15

BREAKFAST:

1 large orange, 2 medium kiwi, or 3 bite-size prunes

1/4 cup whole grain or bran cereal

3/4 cup reduced fat (1%) milk

1 slice whole wheat / whole grain bread, toasted (if desired) with

1 oz reduced fat cheese

Coffee or tea (green or herbal)

MID-MORNING SNACK:

Low-fat fruit-flavored yogurt (6 oz)

_____

LUNCH:

Slimmer Salad Platter (with egg) (page 142)

MID-AFTERNOON SNACK:

2 fruit selections of choice

_____

DINNER:

Chicken and Onion Ragout (page 153)

3/4 cup brown rice

Large tossed salad

BEDTIME SNACK:

6 oz reduced fat (1%) milk or yogurt

DAY 16

BREAKFAST:

1 large orange, 2 medium kiwi, or 3 bite-size prunes

1/4 cup whole grain or bran cereal

3/4 cup reduced fat (1%) milk

1 slice whole wheat / whole grain bread, toasted (if desired) with

3 Tablespoons low-fat cottage cheese

Coffee or tea (green or herbal)

MID-MORNING SNACK:

Low-fat fruit-flavored yogurt (6 oz)

LUNCH:

Chicken and Onion Ragout (from Day 15 dinner; page 153)

Large tossed salad

MID-AFTERNOON SNACK:

2 fruit selections of choice

DINNER:

Fettuccine with Creamy Yogurt Sauce (page 163)

Large tossed salad

BEDTIME SNACK:

6 oz reduced fat (1%) milk or yogurt

DAY 17

BREAKFAST:

1 large orange, 2 medium kiwi, or 3 bite-size prunes

1/4 cup whole grain or bran cereal

3/4 cup reduced fat (1%) milk

1 slice whole wheat / whole grain bread, toasted (if desired) with

2 slices turkey bacon

Coffee or tea (green or herbal)

MID-MORNING SNACK:

Low-fat fruit-flavored yogurt (6 oz)

LUNCH:

Marinated Vegetable Salad (page 143)

1/2 medium whole wheat pita

MID-AFTERNOON SNACK:

Fruit salad with yogurt

DINNER:

Lemon Sole with Parsley Sauce (page 160)

Large tossed salad

BEDTIME SNACK:

6 oz reduced fat (1%) milk or yogurt

DAY 18

It's a Free Day!

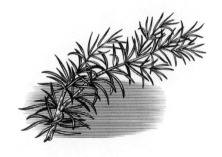

DAY 19

BREAKFAST:

1 large orange, 2 medium kiwi, or 3 bite-size prunes

1/4 cup whole grain or bran cereal

3/4 cup reduced fat (1%) milk

1 slice whole wheat / whole grain bread, toasted (if desired) with

2 small turkey sausages

Coffee or tea (green or herbal)

MID-MORNING SNACK:

Low-fat fruit-flavored yogurt (6 oz)

LUNCH:

Slimmer Salad Platter (with tuna) (page 142)

MID-AFTERNOON SNACK:

1 cup red fruit (choose from cherries, red grapes, or strawberries)

DINNER:

Penne with Grilled Chicken and Pesto (page 154)

Large tossed salad

BEDTIME SNACK:

6 oz reduced fat (1%) milk or yogurt

DAY 20

BREAKFAST:

1 large orange, 2 medium kiwi, or 3 bite-size prunes

1/4 cup whole grain or bran cereal

3/4 cup reduced fat (1%) milk

1 slice whole wheat / whole grain bread, toasted (if desired) with

2 tsp fruit jam or honey

Coffee or tea (green or herbal)

MID-MORNING SNACK:

Low-fat fruit-flavored yogurt (6 oz)

LUNCH:

Mediterranean Chickpea Salad (page 144)

MID-AFTERNOON SNACK:

2 fruit selections of choice

DINNER:

Turkey Meatballs in Tomato Garlic Sauce (page 155)

3/4 cup whole wheat couscous

Large tossed salad

BEDTIME SNACK:

6 oz reduced fat (1%) milk or yogurt

DAY 21

Choose any day's menu from Cycle A or B or have a FREE DAY! (See page 29 to read all about Free Days.)

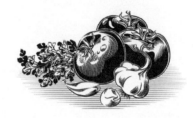

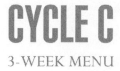

CYCLE C
3-WEEK MENU

DAY 1

BREAKFAST:

1 large orange, 2 medium kiwi, or 3 bite-size prunes

1/4 cup whole grain or bran cereal

3/4 cup reduced fat (1%) milk

1 slice whole wheat / whole grain bread, toasted (if desired) with

1 oz reduced fat cheese

Coffee or tea (green or herbal)

MID-MORNING SNACK:

Low-fat fruit-flavored yogurt (6 oz)

LUNCH:

Tuna Salad with Citronette Dressing (page 167)

2 thin breadsticks or rye crackers

MID-AFTERNOON SNACK:

Fruit salad with yogurt

DINNER:

Mediterranean Chicken Fricasseé (page 177)

Large tossed salad

BEDTIME SNACK:

6 oz reduced fat (1%) milk or plain yogurt

DAY 2

BREAKFAST:

1 large orange, 2 medium kiwi, or 3 bite-size prunes

1/4 cup whole grain or bran cereal

3/4 cup reduced fat (1%) milk

1 slice whole wheat / whole grain bread, toasted (if desired) with

2 tsp fruit jam or honey

Coffee or tea (green or herbal)

MID-MORNING SNACK:

Low-fat fruit-flavored yogurt (6 oz)

LUNCH:

Mediterranean Chicken Fricasseé (from Day 1 dinner; page 177)

1 small whole grain roll

Large tossed salad

MID-AFTERNOON SNACK:

1 cup red fruit (choose from cherries, red grapes, or strawberries)

DINNER:

Veal Scallopini with Quick Caper Sauce (page 183)

Large tossed salad

BEDTIME SNACK:

6 oz reduced fat (1%) milk or yogurt

DAY 3

BREAKFAST:

1 large orange, 2 medium kiwi, or 3 bite-size prunes

1/4 cup whole grain or bran cereal

3/4 cup reduced fat (1%) milk

1 slice whole wheat / whole grain bread, toasted (if desired) with

1 boiled or poached egg

Coffee or tea (green or herbal)

MID-MORNING SNACK:

Low-fat fruit-flavored yogurt (6 oz)

LUNCH:

Lentil Walnut Salad (page 168)

MID-AFTERNOON SNACK:

2 fruit selections of choice

DINNER:

Grilled Chicken Pizza (page 175)

Large tossed salad

BEDTIME SNACK:

6 oz reduced fat (1%) milk or yogurt

DAY 4

BREAKFAST:

1 large orange, 2 medium kiwi, or 3 bite-size prunes

1/4 cup whole grain or bran cereal

3/4 cup reduced fat (1%) milk

1 slice whole wheat / whole grain bread, toasted (if desired) with

1 oz reduced fat cheese

Coffee or tea (green or herbal)

MID-MORNING SNACK:

Low-fat fruit-flavored yogurt (6 oz)

LUNCH:

Deluxe Garden Salad (page 172)

MID-AFTERNOON SNACK:

Orange Chocolate Crunch Cup (page 192)

DINNER:

Slimmer Pasta Alfredo (page 190)

Large tossed salad

BEDTIME SNACK:

6 oz reduced fat (1%) milk or yogurt

DAY 5

BREAKFAST:

1 large orange, 2 medium kiwi, or 3 bite-size prunes

1/4 cup whole grain or bran cereal

3/4 cup reduced fat (1%) milk

1 slice whole wheat / whole grain bread, toasted (if desired) with

2 slices turkey bacon

Coffee or tea (green or herbal)

MID-MORNING SNACK:

Low-fat fruit-flavored yogurt (6 oz)

LUNCH:

Slimmer Caesar Salad with Grilled Chicken (page 169)

2 thin breadsticks or rye crackers

MID-AFTERNOON SNACK:

2 fruit selections of choice

DINNER:

Poached Salmon with Root Vegetables (pages 185-6)

Large tossed salad

BEDTIME SNACK:

6 oz reduced fat (1%) milk or yogurt

DAY 6

BREAKFAST:

1 large orange, 2 medium kiwi, or 3 bite-size prunes

1/4 cup whole grain or bran cereal

3/4 cup reduced fat (1%) milk

1 slice whole wheat / whole grain bread, toasted (if desired) with

2 small turkey sausages

Coffee or tea (green or herbal)

MID-MORNING SNACK:

Low-fat fruit-flavored yogurt (6 oz)

LUNCH:

Poached Salmon Salad Niçoise (page 170)

MID-AFTERNOON SNACK:

1 cup red fruit (choose from cherries, red grapes, or strawberries)

DINNER:

Turkey Phyllo Pot Pie (page 180)

Large tossed salad

BEDTIME SNACK:

6 oz reduced fat (1%) milk or yogurt

DAY 7

Choose any day's menu from Cycle A , B, or C, or have a FREE DAY! (See page 29 to read all about Free Days.)

DAY 8

BREAKFAST:

1 large orange, 2 medium kiwi, or 3 bite-size prunes

1/4 cup whole grain or bran cereal

3/4 cup reduced fat (1%) milk

1 slice whole wheat / whole grain bread, toasted (if desired) with

1 oz reduced fat cheese

Coffee or tea (green or herbal)

MID-MORNING SNACK:

Low-fat fruit-flavored yogurt (6 oz)

LUNCH:

Mediterranean Seafood Salad (page 171)

MID-AFTERNOON SNACK:

Fruit salad with yogurt

DINNER:

Summer Vegetable Risotto with Chicken (page 179)

Large tossed salad

BEDTIME SNACK:

6 oz reduced fat (1%) milk or yogurt

DAY 9

BREAKFAST:

1 large orange, 2 medium kiwi, or 3 bite-size prunes

1/4 cup whole grain or bran cereal

3/4 cup reduced fat (1%) milk

1 slice whole wheat / whole grain bread, toasted (if desired) with

2 tsp fruit jam or honey

Coffee or tea (green or herbal)

MID-MORNING SNACK:

Low-fat fruit-flavored yogurt (6 oz)

LUNCH:

Summer Vegetable Risotto with Chicken (from Day 8 dinner; page 179)

Large tossed salad

MID-AFTERNOON SNACK:

2 fruit selections of choice

DINNER:

Florentine Beef Burger (page 182)

Large tossed salad

BEDTIME SNACK:

6 oz reduced fat (1%) milk or yogurt

DAY 10

BREAKFAST:

1 large orange, 2 medium kiwi, or 3 bite-size prunes

1/4 cup whole grain or bran cereal

3/4 cup reduced fat (1%) milk

1 slice whole wheat / whole grain bread, toasted (if desired) with

2 slices turkey bacon

Coffee or tea (green or herbal)

MID-MORNING SNACK:

Low-fat fruit-flavored yogurt (6 oz)

LUNCH:

Florentine Beef Burger (from Day 9 dinner; page 182)

Large tossed salad

MID-AFTERNOON SNACK:

1 cup red fruit (choose from cherries, red grapes, or strawberries)

DINNER:

Sausage and Peppers with Orzo (page 184)

Large tossed salad

BEDTIME SNACK:

6 oz reduced fat (1%) milk or yogurt

DAY 11

BREAKFAST:

1 large orange, 2 medium kiwi, or 3 bite-size prunes

1/4 cup whole grain or bran cereal

3/4 cup reduced fat (1%) milk

1 slice whole wheat / whole grain bread, toasted (if desired) with

3 Tablespoons low-fat cottage cheese and

2 small turkey sausages

Coffee or tea (green or herbal)

MID-MORNING SNACK:

Low-fat fruit-flavored yogurt (6 oz)

LUNCH:

Deluxe Garden Salad (page 172)

MID-AFTERNOON SNACK:

Fruit salad with yogurt

DINNER:

Greek Olympiad Pizza (page 174)

Large tossed salad

BEDTIME SNACK:

6 oz reduced fat (1%) milk or yogurt

DAY 12

BREAKFAST:

1 large orange, 2 medium kiwi, or 3 bite-size prunes

1/4 cup whole grain or bran cereal

3/4 cup reduced fat (1%) milk

1 slice whole wheat / whole grain bread, toasted (if desired) with

2 small turkey sausages

Coffee or tea (green or herbal)

MID-MORNING SNACK:

Low-fat fruit-flavored yogurt (6 oz)

LUNCH:

Slimmer Chef's Salad (page 105)

2 breadsticks or rye crackers

MID-AFTERNOON SNACK:

1 cup red fruit (choose from cherries, red grapes, or strawberries)

DINNER:

Greek-style Grilled Fish and Vegetables (page 189)

Large tossed salad

BEDTIME SNACK:

6 oz reduced fat (1%) milk or yogurt

DAY 13

BREAKFAST:

1 large orange, 2 medium kiwi, or 3 bite-size prunes

1/4 cup whole grain or bran cereal

3/4 cup reduced fat (1%) milk

1 slice whole wheat / whole grain bread, toasted (if desired) with

2 slices turkey bacon

Coffee or tea (green or herbal)

MID-MORNING SNACK:

Low-fat fruit-flavored yogurt (6 oz)

LUNCH:

Shrimp with Garlic Aioli (page 173)

Large tossed salad

MID-AFTERNOON SNACK:

2 fruit selections of choice

DINNER:

Chicken with Yogurt Sauce (page 178)

3/4 cup brown rice

Large tossed salad

BEDTIME SNACK:

6 oz reduced fat (1%) milk or yogurt

DAY 14

Choose any day's menu from Cycle A, B, or C, or have a FREE DAY! (See page 29 to read all about Free Days.)

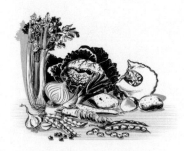

DAY 15

BREAKFAST:

1 large orange, 2 medium kiwi, or 3 bite-size prunes

1/4 cup whole grain or bran cereal

3/4 cup reduced fat (1%) milk

1 slice whole wheat / whole grain bread, toasted (if desired) with

1 oz reduced fat cheese

Coffee or tea (green or herbal)

MID-MORNING SNACK:

Low-fat fruit-flavored yogurt (6 oz)

LUNCH:

Chicken with Yogurt Sauce (from Day 13 dinner; page 178)

1/2 medium whole wheat pita

Large tossed salad

MID-AFTERNOON SNACK:

2 fruit selections of choice

DINNER:

Baked Cod Casserole (page 188)

Large tossed salad

BEDTIME SNACK:

6 oz reduced fat (1%) milk or yogurt

DAY 16

BREAKFAST:

1 large orange, 2 medium kiwi, or 3 bite-size prunes

1/4 cup whole grain or bran cereal

3/4 cup reduced fat (1%) milk

1 slice whole wheat / whole grain bread, toasted (if desired) with

3 Tablespoons low-fat cottage cheese

Coffee or tea (green or herbal)

MID-MORNING SNACK:

Low-fat fruit-flavored yogurt (6 oz)

LUNCH:

Baked Cod Casserole (from Day 15 dinner; page 188)

Large tossed salad

MID-AFTERNOON SNACK:

2 fruit selections of choice

DINNER:

Beef and Mushroom Ragout (page 181)

3/4 cup brown rice

Large tossed salad

BEDTIME SNACK:

6 oz reduced fat (1%) milk or yogurt

DAY 17

BREAKFAST:

1 large orange, 2 medium kiwi, or 3 bite-size prunes

1/4 cup whole grain or bran cereal

3/4 cup reduced fat (1%) milk

1 slice whole wheat / whole grain bread, toasted (if desired) with

2 slices turkey bacon

Coffee or tea (green or herbal)

MID-MORNING SNACK:

Low-fat fruit-flavored yogurt (6 oz)

LUNCH:

Beef and Mushroom Ragout (from Day 16 dinner; page 181)

3/4 cup brown rice

Large tossed salad

MID-AFTERNOON SNACK:

1 cup red fruit (choose from cherries, red grapes, or strawberries)

DINNER:

Baked Salmon with Fennel and Tomatoes (page 187)

Large tossed salad

BEDTIME SNACK:

6 oz reduced fat (1%) milk or yogurt

DAY 18

BREAKFAST:

1 large orange, 2 medium kiwi, or 3 bite-size prunes

1/4 cup whole grain or bran cereal

3/4 cup reduced fat (1%) milk

1 slice whole wheat / whole grain bread, toasted (if desired) with

2 tsp fruit jam or honey

Coffee or tea (green or herbal)

MID-MORNING SNACK:

Low-fat fruit-flavored yogurt (6 oz)

LUNCH:

Baked Salmon with Fennel and Tomatoes (from Day 17 dinner; page 187)

Large tossed salad

MID-AFTERNOON SNACK:

2 fruit selections of choice

DINNER:

Chickpea Curry Stew (page 191)

3/4 cup whole wheat couscous

Large tossed salad

BEDTIME SNACK:

6 oz reduced fat (1%) milk or yogurt

DAY 19

BREAKFAST:

1 large orange, 2 medium kiwi, or 3 bite-size prunes

1/4 cup whole grain or bran cereal

3/4 cup reduced fat (1%) milk

1 slice whole wheat / whole grain bread, toasted (if desired) with

2 small turkey sausages

Coffee or tea (green or herbal)

MID-MORNING SNACK:

Low-fat fruit-flavored yogurt (6 oz)

LUNCH:

Chickpea Curry Stew (from Day 18 dinner; page 191)

Large tossed salad

MID-AFTERNOON SNACK:

1 cup red fruit (choose from cherries, red grapes, or strawberries)

DINNER:

Whole Wheat Baguette Pizza (page 176)

Large tossed salad

BEDTIME SNACK:

6 oz reduced fat (1%) milk or yogurt

DAY 20

It's a Free Day!

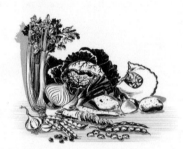

DAY 21

Choose any day's menu from Cycle A, B, or C, or have a FREE DAY! (See page 29 to read all about Free Days.)

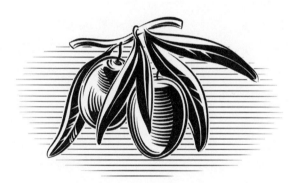

The Recipes

CYCLE A

Slimmer Chef's Salad

Slimmer Greek Salad

Salmon Salad with Honey and Balsamic Dressing

Mediterranean Tuna Salad

Slimmer Egg Salad Pita

Pasta Salad Primavera

Tomato and Lentil Soup

Three Bean Soup

Pepperoni Pita Pizza with Marinara Sauce

Slimmer Greek Salad Pizza

Slimmer Chicken à la Crème

Greek Chicken with Roast Potatoes

Chicken Stew with Garden Peas

Spaghetti Bolognese

Mediterranean Burger

Greek-style Sliders with Yogurt Sauce

Beefsteak Florentine

Veal or Pork Provençal

Sole with Oregano and Lemon

Baked Fish and Vegetables Aegean Style

Shrimp with Lemon Sauce

Easy Seafood Risotto

Mediterranean Mac and Cheese

Pasta Puttanesca

Slimmer Loaded Baked Potato

Slimmer Fruit Salad

Fruit Salad with Yogurt Crunch

Cinnamon Apple Greek Yogurt

Banana Walnut Yogurt

Pear and Yogurt Parfait

Slimmer Chef's Salad

This chef's salad with a healthy twist is a perfect packed lunch for work. Bring your dressing in a separate container to pour just before serving.

2 cups bite-size Romaine lettuce leaves
1/2 medium tomato, sliced
1/2 cup sliced cucumber
1/4 cup carrot, shredded
1 hard-boiled egg, sliced
1 oz sliced turkey breast
1 oz sliced reduced fat cheese, such as Swiss or Munster

For the dressing:
2 Tablespoons nonfat plain Greek yogurt
2 teaspoons low-fat mayonnaise
1 teaspoon cocktail sauce
A dash of balsamic vinegar or lemon juice
Salt and pepper to taste

1. Toss together the lettuce, tomato, cucumber, and carrot, and place in a serving bowl. Arrange the egg over the top. Place the turkey on top of the cheese slice, roll into a "cigar" and cut spiral slices, adding to the top. Cover and keep refrigerated until ready to eat.
2. In a small bowl or container stir together the dressing ingredients and keep refrigerated until ready to serve.

Makes 1 serving

Slimmer Greek Salad

A popular order at Maria and Eleni's Taverna, this updated version of a classic American favorite is abounding in the flavors of Greece. Bring your dressing in a separate container for workday lunch and pour just before serving.

2 cups Mediterranean greens such as escarole,
   romaine, and radicchio
1/4 cup cherry or grape tomatoes
1/4 cup sliced cucumber
1/4 cup sliced green bell pepper
2 Tablespoons shaved red onion
2 or 3 Kalamata olives
1 oz crumbled feta cheese

For the dressing:
2 teaspoons olive oil
A drizzle of balsamic vinegar
A pinch of dried oregano
Salt and pepper to taste

1. Toss together the greens, tomatoes, cucumber, bell pepper, and onion, and place in a serving bowl. Top with the olives and cheese.
2. In a small bowl or container stir together the dressing ingredients and pour on salad just before serving.

Makes 1 serving

Salmon Salad with Honey and Balsamic Dressing

Smoked salmon stars in this colorful salad with a slightly sweet dressing. You could also use flaked poached salmon or drained, canned Alaskan salmon for variety.

2 cups mixed salad greens
1/4 cup shredded red cabbage
1 scallion, trimmed and sliced
2 Tablespoons shredded carrot
2 sundried tomato pieces, sliced
2 oz smoked salmon, cut into pieces

For the dressing:
1 teaspoon prepared mustard
1 teaspoon honey
2 teaspoons balsamic vinegar
2 teaspoons olive oil
Salt and pepper to taste

1. Combine the salad ingredients in a serving bowl or airtight container, if bringing to work, and toss gently. Keep refrigerated until ready to eat.
2. In a separate bowl or container whisk together the dressing ingredients and keep refrigerated.
3. When ready to serve, pour the dressing over and toss gently to coat.

Makes 1 serving

Mediterranean Tuna Salad

A welcome and healthier version of typical tuna salad, this Mediterranean-style lunch is great for bringing to work. Pack the dressing
separately and add just before eating.

2 cups mixed salad greens
1/2 small cucumber, sliced
1/2 small green bell pepper, cored, seeded, and diced
1 Tablespoon chopped fresh dill sprigs
1/4 cup grape tomatoes
One small can solid tuna packed in water,
    well-drained and flaked
1/4 cup canned cannellini beans, drained and rinsed

For the dressing:
Juice of 1/2 a lemon
1 teaspoon prepared mustard
2 teaspoons olive oil
Salt and pepper to taste

Combine the salad ingredients in a serving bowl or an
airtight container and refrigerate until ready to eat. In
a separate bowl or container, stir together the dressing
ingredients and refrigerate. Dress and toss the salad just
before serving.

Makes 1 serving

Slimmer Egg Salad Pita

Creamy and delicious egg salad is the perfect filling for a pita pocket. This version will delight you with the tang of mustard and the addition of feta cheese.

2 large hard-boiled eggs (1 yolk only)
Salt and pepper to taste
2 teaspoons low-fat mayonnaise
1/2 teaspoon prepared mustard
1 Tablespoon crumbled feta cheese
1 teaspoon chopped fresh parsley

1/2 medium whole wheat pita

Place the eggs in a small bowl and, using the back of a fork, mash them to desired consistency. Stir in the remaining ingredients and fill the pita with the mixture. Wrap and refrigerate until ready to eat or serve immediately.

Makes 1 serving

Pasta Salad Primavera

Any type of pasta shape will do in this satisfying salad that's full of nutrition. Try substituting flaked tuna, diced chicken breast, or baby shrimp for the turkey.

1 1/2 cups cooked small pasta shells
1 Tablespoon finely chopped onion
2 Tablespoons diced green bell pepper
2 Tablespoons shredded carrot
1/2 medium tomato, seeded and chopped
1/2 small cucumber, diced
1/2 cup cooked broccoli florets
1 oz cooked turkey breast, diced

For the dressing:
2 Tablespoons nonfat plain Greek yogurt
2 teaspoons low-fat mayonnaise
1 teaspoon cocktail sauce
1 teaspoon prepared mustard
Salt and pepper to taste

1. Place all the salad ingredients in a bowl and toss to combine.
2. Make the dressing by stirring together the ingredients in a small bowl, and then pour over the salad. Stir gently to coat all the ingredients, taste for additional seasoning, and serve or refrigerate until ready to eat.

Makes 1 serving

Tomato and Lentil Soup

Hearty and satisfying, this nutritious soup can be easily doubled for another day's lunch or Free Day meal.

2 teaspoons olive oil
I small onion, finely chopped
I small carrot, finely chopped
Salt and pepper to taste
I garlic clove, minced
2/3 cup dry lentils, rinsed
I cup water
I bay leaf
1/4 teaspoon dried oregano
I cup crushed tomatoes
A dash of balsamic vinegar

1. Heat the oil in a medium saucepan over medium heat. Add the onion and carrot, season with salt and pepper, and cook, stirring occasionally, until the vegetables are slightly softened, about 2 minutes. Add the garlic and cook 1 minute more.

2. Stir in the lentils, water, bay leaf, and oregano. Bring to a simmer, reduce the heat to low, and cook for 15 minutes until the lentils are tender but firm. Stir occasionally and add a touch more water if necessary to prevent sticking.

3. Add the crushed tomatoes and continue cooking until the lentils are softened and the soup is thick and rich, about 8 minutes more. Remove the bay leaf, taste for seasoning, and finish with the dash of vinegar.

Makes 1 serving

Three Bean Soup

You'll love the creamy richness of this soup, which can be easily doubled or tripled for other lunches or Free Days meals.

2 teaspoons olive oil
1/2 small onion, diced
1/2 small carrot, diced
1/2 small celery stalk, diced
Salt and pepper to taste
2/3 cup canned chickpeas, drained and rinsed
1/3 cup each canned red or
   white kidney beans, and Borlotti beans, drained, and rinsed
1 1/2 cups low-sodium chicken broth
1/4 teaspoon dried thyme
A few drops of lemon juice

1. Heat the oil in a medium saucepan over medium-high heat. Add the onion, carrot, and celery, season with salt and pepper, and cook, stirring often, until the vegetables are tender, about 6 minutes.
2. Add the remaining ingredients except the lemon juice, bring to a simmer, and cook over low heat for 5 minutes.
3. Remove from the heat and using a handheld immersion blender or a potato masher, blend the soup to thicken, keeping about half the beans intact. Stir in the lemon juice and serve.

Makes 1 serving

Pepperoni Pita Pizza

You can also prepare this pizza using a whole grain pre-baked individual-size pizza base following the heating directions on the packaging. For homemade marinara sauce, see directions on the following page.

1 medium or 2 small whole wheat pitas
2 Tablespoons prepared marinara sauce
3 Tablespoons shredded reduced fat mozzarella
1 oz sliced turkey pepperoni

1. Preheat the oven to 350° F. Place a baking sheet in the oven while heating.
2. Spread the sauce on top of the pitas, sprinkle with the cheese, and place the pepperoni evenly over the top.
3. Bake the pitas in the oven on the baking sheet until the bottom is somewhat crispy and the cheese has melted, 10 to 12 minutes.

Makes 1 serving

Slimmer Marinara Sauce

2 cups chopped fresh or canned tomatoes
1 Tablespoon tomato paste
1 Tablespoon olive oil
2 teaspoons balsamic vinegar
1 small garlic clove, minced
Salt and freshly ground pepper to taste
1 teaspoon dried basil
1 teaspoon dried oregano

1. Combine all the ingredients except the herbs in a medium saucepan. Bring to a simmer over medium heat, stirring often.
2. Reduce the heat to low and cook, stirring occasionally, 10 to 12 minutes. Add the herbs and cook a further 3 to 5 minutes. Taste for seasoning and set aside to cool slightly.
3. Blend on low in an immersion blender or food processor just until smooth. The sauce can be frozen in a tightly sealed container for up to 3 months.

Makes about 1 1/2 cups

Slimmer Greek Salad Pizza

A variation on a wonderful dish served at Maria and Eleni's Taverna, this selection is the perfect dinner when Greek Salad is on tomorrow's lunch menu. Make half a recipe extra and get two meals in one!

1 individual pre-baked pizza crust
1 Tablespoon marinara sauce (for homemade, see p. 114)
1/2 recipe Slimmer Greek Salad (p. 106),
    olives and feta set aside

1. Preheat the oven according to pizza crust directions. Place the crust on a baking sheet and spread the sauce over. Chop the olives and sprinkle them with the crumbled feta over the sauce.
2. Bake according to package instructions until the cheese melts and the pizza is well heated and crisp on the edges, about 12 minutes. Remove from the oven and transfer to a serving dish.
3. Toss the salad with the dressing in a medium bowl and pile on top of the cooked pizza. Serve immediately.

Makes 1 serving

Slimmer Pizza Dough

3 1/3 cups all-purpose flour, or more for kneading
1/2 packet dry yeast
1 teaspoon cornstarch
1/2 teaspoon organic sugar
A pinch of salt
2 teaspoons olive oil
1/2 cup warm water

1. Place the flour in a large bowl and make a hollow in the center. Add the yeast, cornstarch, sugar, salt, olive oil, and most but not all of the water.
2. Stir together with your fingers and form into a ball. Add water or flour as needed to keep its shape.
3. Transfer to a floured board and knead until the dough is smooth and no longer sticks to your hands, about 3 to 5 minutes.
4. Divide into 9 equal portions, shape into disks, wrap with plastic, and refrigerate or freeze until ready to use.

Slimmer Chicken à la Crème

Unbelievably rich and creamy, this dish is sure to satisfy any appetite. Try serving with rice for dinner and then serving your lunch portion in half a whole wheat pita pocket.

I teaspoon olive oil
2 boneless, skinless chicken breasts, cut into I-inch cubes
Salt and pepper to taste
I small onion, finely chopped
I cup thinly sliced white mushrooms
3 Tablespoons dry white wine
I cup low-sodium chicken broth or water
1/2 cup low-fat evaporated milk
2 teaspoons prepared mustard
I teaspoon cornstarch

1. Heat the oil in a large nonstick pan over medium-high heat. Season the chicken with salt and pepper and cook in the oil, stirring frequently to lightly brown, about 2 minutes. Transfer with a slotted spoon to a plate and set aside.

2. Add the onion and mushrooms to the skillet and cook, stirring often, until somewhat softened and lightly browned, about 4 minutes. Return the chicken with its juices to the pan and add the wine. Stir well and cook for 1 minute over high heat. Add the broth, bring to a simmer, cover, reduce the heat to low, and cook until the chicken is firm and no longer pink inside, about 10 minutes.

3. In a small bowl whisk together the milk, mustard, and cornstarch. Stir the mixture into the pan and bring to a simmer. Continue cooking for 2 minutes until the sauce is thick and rich. Taste for seasoning and serve immediately.

Makes 2 servings

Greek Chicken with Roast Potatoes

Roasting brings out the flavor in this one-dish meal featuring the piquancy of citrus and the aroma of fresh herbs.

2 medium split chicken breasts, skin removed and
   trimmed of fat
Salt and pepper to taste
2 medium red or Yukon Gold potatoes, cubed
2 garlic cloves, smashed
2/3 cup water
Juice of 1 lemon
Juice of 1/2 an orange
2 teaspoons olive oil
1 teaspoon prepared mustard
1 sprig fresh rosemary
1 sprig fresh oregano

1. Preheat the oven to 375° F.
2. Season the chicken breasts and place flesh side down in the middle of a nonstick roasting pan. Distribute the potatoes and garlic around.
3. In a small bowl whisk together the water, lemon and orange juice, oil, and mustard and pour into the pan, stirring to distribute. Add the herbs and roast in the oven, occasionally stirring to evenly cook and brown, until the potatoes are tender, the liquid has evaporated, and an instant-read thermometer reaches 165° F when inserted in the chicken breast.
4. Remove from the oven and allow to rest for 5 minutes before serving.

Makes 2 servings

Chicken Stew with Garden Peas

Lots of flavor and healthy fiber highlight this stew that tastes even better the next day!

I Tablespoon olive oil, plus I additional teaspoon set aside
I medium onion, finely diced
2 scallions, trimmed and diced
8 oz boneless, skinless chicken, cut into I-inch cubes
Salt and pepper to taste
2 cups frozen garden peas
1/2 small carrot, thinly sliced
One 8 oz can tomato sauce
I cup low-sodium chicken broth or water
2 teaspoons chopped fresh dill

1. Heat the tablespoon of oil in a nonstick pot over medium-high heat. Add the onion, scallions, and chicken cubes, season with salt and pepper, and cook, stirring often, until the onion is softened and the chicken is no longer pink, about 4 minutes.
2. Stir in the peas and carrot and cook a further minute. Pour in the tomato sauce and broth, stir well to combine, and bring to a simmer. Reduce the heat to low and cook until the vegetables are tender and the stew is thickened, about 15 minutes.
3. Remove from the heat and stir in the remaining olive oil and dill.

Makes 2 servings

Spaghetti Bolognese

Enjoy this lighter version of a Mediterranean classic that's almost as quick to make as it is to eat. Don't skimp on good quality Parmesan to finish it off.

1 teaspoon olive oil
1 small onion, finely chopped
1/4 cup finely chopped green bell pepper
1/2 cup thinly sliced white mushrooms
4 oz lean ground beef
Salt and pepper to taste
2 Tablespoons dry white wine
One 8 oz can tomato sauce
1 teaspoon tomato paste
1 small cinnamon stick
A pinch of ground allspice
2/3 cup water
1/2 teaspoon finely chopped parsley leaves
1 Tablespoon nonfat Greek yogurt (optional)
2 oz spaghetti, cooked according to package instructions
1 Tablespoon grated Parmesan cheese to serve

1. Heat the oil in a large nonstick pan over medium-high heat, add the onion, green pepper, mushrooms, and beef, season with salt and pepper, and cook, using a fork to break up the meat, until the beef is browned and the vegetables are softened, 6 to 8 minutes. Add the wine and cook a further minute.
2. Stir in the tomato sauce and paste and add the cinnamon and allspice. Cook the mixture while stirring for an additional minute. Pour in the water, bring to a simmer, cover, and cook over low heat until the mixture is thick and well blended, 10 to 12 minutes. Add the parsley and yogurt, if using. Stir well to combine, and cook 2 minutes more.
3. Add the cooked spaghetti to the pan, toss well to coat and heat through. Serve topped with the Parmesan.

Makes 1 serving

Mediterranean Burger

This healthy rendition of everyone's favorite is surprisingly hearty and flavorful without the usual bun and condiments. Try making it with lean ground lamb when available, adding a pinch of chopped fresh mint.

4 oz lean ground beef
Salt and pepper to taste
1 Tablespoon flaxseed meal
1 Tablespoon ground oats *
1 Tablespoon finely chopped sundried tomato
1 small garlic clove, minced
1/4 teaspoon onion flakes
1/4 teaspoon dried parsley
A dash of balsamic vinegar

For burger sauce:
Juice of 1/2 a lemon
2 teaspoons olive oil
1 teaspoon prepared mustard
A pinch of dried oregano
Salt and pepper to taste

1. Combine all the burger ingredients in a small bowl and shape into a patty. Whisk together the sauce ingredients in a small bowl and set aside.
2. Heat a nonstick skillet or grill over medium-high heat and cook the burger on both sides, until firm to the touch and no longer pink inside, about 8 minutes total.
3. Transfer the burger to a serving dish and immediately pour the sauce over the burger.

* Make ground oats by pulverizing old-fashioned oatmeal flakes in a blender or food processor.

Makes 1 serving

Greek-style Sliders with Yogurt Sauce

These two-bite burgers are great for hearty appetites at lunch or dinner and could also be made with ground beef or turkey, if preferred.

8 oz lean ground lamb
Salt and pepper to taste
1/2 medium onion, finely chopped
1 garlic clove, minced
2 Tablespoons flaxseed meal
1 Tablespoon ground oats
1 teaspoon prepared mustard
1/4 teaspoon dried oregano

For the yogurt sauce:
1/4 cup nonfat plain Greek yogurt
1/2 teaspoon each: finely chopped fresh mint and parsley
1 teaspoon fresh lemon juice
2 Tablespoons diced cucumber

To serve:
6 miniature whole wheat pitas
1/2 medium tomato, seeded and diced

1. In a medium bowl combine the burger ingredients, mixing well. Form into 6 patties, cover, and refrigerate until ready to cook.
2. In a small bowl combine the sauce ingredients and refrigerate.
3. Heat a grill or broiler and cook the patties until nicely browned and no longer pink inside, about 3 minutes per side.
4. To serve, insert the burger into the pita pocket, and top with a small dollop of the sauce and a little of the tomato.

Makes 2 servings

Beefsteak Florentine

A quick sauté of spinach as a bed turns this tender steak into a dinner treat in the style of Florence. Serve with whole grain bread to soak up the delicious juices.

I teaspoon olive oil
2 cups baby spinach leaves
I garlic clove, minced
Salt and pepper to taste
One 4 oz thin-cut boneless sirloin steak, trimmed of all fat
3 Tablespoons dry white wine
I Tablespoon water
I teaspoon prepared mustard
Lemon wedge for serving

1. Heat the oil in a large nonstick skillet over medium heat. Add the spinach leaves and gently toss until the volume is reduced by half, about 1 minute. Add the garlic, salt, and pepper, and continue cooking until wilted and tender, about 2 minutes more. Transfer to a serving plate and set aside to keep warm.

2. Season the steak with salt and pepper and brown in the skillet over high heat on both sides, about 3 minutes each. Combine the remaining ingredients except for the lemon, and pour over the steak.

3. Reduce the heat and cook, covered, to desired doneness, about 3 minutes for medium. Place the steak on top of the cooked spinach, pour the sauce over, and serve with the lemon wedge.

Makes 1 serving

Veal or Pork Provençal

Cooking in a foil packet makes cleanup a breeze. Try this method with fish fillets such as salmon, halibut, or cod.

4 oz thin-cut veal or pork scaloppini
Salt and pepper to taste
1/4 cup thinly sliced onion
1/2 cup thinly sliced red, orange, or green bell pepper
1 plum tomato, sliced
A splash of white wine or apple juice
A pinch of dried Herbes de Provence

1. Preheat the oven to 350° F. Place a rimmed baking sheet in the oven while heating.
2. Place a 12-inch piece of foil on a flat surface and fan out the veal/pork in the middle. Sprinkle with salt and pepper. Place the vegetables evenly on top, add the wine and herbs, and close up the foil into an airtight tent shape.
3. Place on the heated baking sheet and cook for 20 to 25 minutes. You can carefully open the packet to check that the veal/pork is no longer pink.
4. Open the packet on the baking sheet and briefly turn on the broiler just to lightly brown, for 2 to 3 minutes. Serve immediately.

Makes 1 serving

Note: Herbes de Provence is a classic blend of 7 French herbs, available in the spice and herb aisle of most supermarkets.

Sole with Oregano and Lemon

This easy preparation highlights the flavor of simple and fresh ingredients reminiscent of the Mediterranean. It is always a popular dish at Maria and Eleni's Taverna.

Four 1 oz sole or flounder fillets
Salt and pepper to taste
Juice of 1/2 a lemon
2 teaspoons olive oil
1 Tablespoon shaved red onion
1/2 teaspoon minced fresh oregano leaves

1. Preheat an oven broiler to high. Line a broiler pan with foil and place the fish fillets in a single layer on the pan. Season with salt and pepper and set aside.
2. In a small bowl combine the remaining ingredients.
3. Broil the fish, turning the pan occasionally to evenly cook, until the fillets are firm and white, 3 to 5 minutes. Using a spatula, carefully transfer the cooked fillets to a serving dish and immediately pour the lemon mixture over.

Makes 1 serving

Baked Fish and Vegetables Aegean Style

Have your fishmonger fillet your snapper or use a boneless, skin-less cod or scrod fillet in this aromatic dish that will take you to the Aegean coast in no time. A variation of the dish is beloved by diners at the Taverna.

2 teaspoons olive oil
8 oz red snapper fish (3 or 4 medium-size fillets)
1 medium garlic clove, roughly chopped
Salt and pepper to taste
1/2 medium onion, thinly sliced
1/2 red bell pepper, seeded and thinly sliced
1/2 medium zucchini, cut into 1/2-inch circles
3 baby carrots, thinly sliced
2 plum tomatoes, roughly chopped
1/4 cup dry white wine
Finely chopped fresh parsley to serve

1. Preheat the oven to 350° F. Drizzle the olive oil in the bottom of a medium-size casserole with a lid. Place the fish in a single layer on the bottom, sprinkle the garlic, salt, and pepper over, and place the onion, pepper, zucchini, carrots, and tomatoes evenly over and around. Sprinkle again with salt and pepper, and drizzle the white wine over all.
2. Cover and bake in the oven, occasionally stirring the vegetables to cook evenly, being careful not to break apart the fish, until they are tender and the fish is cooked through, about 1 hour.
3. Before serving sprinkle with the chopped parsley.

Makes 2 servings

Shrimp with Lemon Sauce

Garlic and lemon provide the tangy flavor in this quick, one-skillet dish featuring jumbo shrimp and broccoli.

1 teaspoon olive oil
1 garlic clove, minced
Salt and pepper to taste
4 oz jumbo shrimp, peeled and deveined
1 cup broccoli florets, steamed to crisp yet tender
1/4 cup vegetable broth or water
Juice of 1 lemon

1. Heat the oil in a nonstick skillet over medium heat. Add the garlic and cook for a few seconds. Season the shrimp with salt and pepper and add to the skillet.
2. Cook, stirring frequently, until the shrimp is pink, about 2 minutes. Add the remaining ingredients, stir well to coat, and cook for 1 minute more. Serve immediately.

Makes 1 serving

Easy Seafood Risotto

No constant stirring required in this easy-to-make version of a favorite Italian rice dish, also a variation of a favorite dish enjoyed at Maria and Eleni's Taverna. You can vary the seafood you select according to availability and substitute another rice if necessary.

2 teaspoons olive oil
I small onion or shallot, minced
I garlic clove, minced
Salt and pepper to taste
I Tablespoon balsamic vinegar
I cup crushed tomatoes
A dash of cayenne pepper
2 cups cooked mixed seafood such as small shrimp, mussels,
   baby scallops, or calamari
2 cups cooked plain Arborio rice, hot
2 teaspoons chopped fresh parsley

1. Heat the oil in a large saucepan over medium heat. Add the onion and garlic, season with salt and pepper and cook, stirring often, for 2 minutes. Add the vinegar and cook a further minute.
2. Stir in the tomatoes and cayenne, bring to a simmer, reduce the heat to low, and cook until thickened and somewhat reduced, about 10 minutes.
3. Add the seafood and continue cooking until heated through, about 3 minutes. Remove from the heat, stir in the rice and parsley, and serve immediately.

Makes 2 servings

Mediterranean Mac and Cheese

Enjoy the richness and creaminess of classic comfort food in this guiltless preparation that's also easy to make.

3/4 cup reduced fat milk
2 teaspoons cornstarch
1 Tablespoon cold water
Salt and pepper to taste
1/3 cup grated Gouda cheese
1 egg, slightly beaten
1 1/2 cups cooked elbow or other small macaroni
1 teaspoon unsalted butter, diced
1 medium tomato, sliced

1. Preheat the oven to 350° F.
2. Heat the milk in a medium saucepan until just scalded. In a small cup stir together the cornstarch and water until smooth. Pour into the hot milk and stir constantly until bubbly and thick, about 2 minutes.
3. Remove from the heat and add the salt, pepper, and cheese. Stir until the cheese has melted, then slowly add the beaten egg.
4. Stir in the macaroni and transfer to a medium glass or ceramic baking dish. Top with the diced butter and the tomato slices and bake until the top is browned and the edges are bubbly, 20 to 30 minutes.

Makes 1 serving

Pasta Puttanesca

This quick and spicy sauce for spaghetti will delight your taste buds with every bite.

2 teaspoons olive oil
I large garlic clove, minced
I anchovy fillet, chopped
I cup canned tomatoes with juice, chopped
I Tablespoon tomato paste
A dash of cayenne pepper
I teaspoon small capers
2 Kalamata olives, pitted and chopped
I teaspoon finely chopped fresh parsley
Salt and pepper to taste
2 oz spaghetti, cooked according to package instructions
I Tablespoon crumbled feta cheese

1. Heat the oil in a medium nonstick pan over medium-high heat. Add the garlic and anchovy and cook, stirring constantly, for 1 minute. Add the tomatoes, paste, cayenne, capers, and olives, stir well to combine, bring to a simmer, and cook over low heat for 5 minutes.
2. Add the parsley and taste for the addition of salt and pepper. Add the cooked spaghetti and toss well to coat, heating until bubbly. Transfer to a serving dish and top with the cheese.

Makes 1 serving

Slimmer Loaded Baked Potato

Dive into this satisfying potato that's loaded with nutrition and perfect when served with a large salad or steamed veggies.

1 large baking potato (Idaho, russet, or Yukon Gold)
1 teaspoon unsalted butter
Salt and pepper to taste
2 Tablespoons nonfat Greek yogurt
1 scallion, trimmed and finely chopped
1 hard-boiled egg, roughly chopped

1. Preheat the oven to 375° F. Poke a few holes in the potato with a fork.
2. Bake the potato in the upper half of the oven until a fork inserted comes out easily and the skin is nicely crisp, about 1 hour.
3. Transfer the potato to a serving dish. Cut down the middle and squeeze the ends together to open. Top with the butter, salt, pepper, and yogurt. Finish with the scallion and chopped egg and serve immediately.

Makes 1 serving

Slimmer Fruit Salad

Although any number of fruits are great for salad making, this combination travels particularly well for work or school and can be prepared the night before.

1/4 cup seedless red grapes
1 small tangerine or Clementine orange, peeled and
   segmented
1/2 cup strawberries, stemmed and halved
1/4 cup blueberries

Combine all the ingredients in an airtight container and keep refrigerated until ready to eat.

Makes 1 serving

Fruit Salad with Yogurt Crunch

This is a delightful snack that's a little bit sweet and perfect for an afternoon break. We even serve it as a light dessert at Maria and Eleni's Taverna. If bringing to work, pack the fruit and yogurt mixture separately and combine just before eating.

For the fruit salad:
1/2 medium apple, cored and diced
I small apricot, pitted and diced
I teaspoon lemon juice
A dash of ground cinnamon
I Tablespoon dried cranberries

For the yogurt crunch:
1/2 cup nonfat or low-fat Greek yogurt
I Tablespoon granola
I Tablespoon chopped walnuts

1. Combine the fruit salad ingredients in an airtight container and keep refrigerated until ready to eat. Also combine the yogurt ingredients in a separate airtight container until ready to eat.
2. To serve, combine both mixtures in a small dish and stir together.

Makes 1 serving

Cinnamon Apple Greek Yogurt

This delicious combination will become a favorite snack. Try different types of locally grown apples depending on the season, such as Pippin and Macintosh.

6 oz nonfat plain Greek yogurt
I medium apple, cored and diced
I Tablespoon golden raisins
A dash of ground cinnamon

Stir together all the ingredients in a small bowl and keep refrigerated until ready to serve.

Makes 1 serving

VARIATIONS:
- *Substitute 1 medium Bosc pear for the apple and 1 chopped date for the raisins.*
- *Substitute 1 Asian pear for the apple and 1 Tablespoon dried goji berries for the raisins.*

Banana Walnut Yogurt

Bring the unpeeled banana with you to work so you can peel and slice when ready to indulge in this terrific snack.

I medium banana, peeled and sliced
1/2 cup low-fat or nonfat plain Greek yogurt
I Tablespoon chopped walnuts
A dash of cinnamon

Place the sliced banana in the bottom of a small bowl and top with the yogurt, nuts, and cinnamon. Serve immediately.

Makes 1 serving

Pear and Yogurt Parfait

The combination of sweet pear and creamy yogurt is a dynamic pairing that can't be beat except when honey and lemon are added!

1 pear, such as Comice, cored and diced
1 teaspoon lemon juice
1/2 cup nonfat Greek yogurt
1/4 teaspoon grated lemon rind
1 teaspoon honey

1. Place the diced pear in a small bowl and gently toss with the lemon juice. Set aside.
2. In a small bowl stir together the yogurt, lemon rind, and honey. Using a parfait or wine goblet, layer the fruit and yogurt mixtures decoratively. Cover and refrigerate or serve immediately.

Makes 1 serving

CYCLE B

Slimmer Shrimp Salad

Slimmer Potato and Egg Salad

Salmon Salad Platter

Slimmer Salad Platter

Marinated Vegetable Salad

Mediterranean Chickpea Salad

Slimmer Club Sandwich

Bean and Vegetable Chowder

White Bean Soup

Slimmer Sausage Pizza

Greek-style Phyllo Calzone

Garden Vegetable Omelette

Chicken with Orzo

Herb Roasted Chicken with Vegetables

Chicken and Onion Ragout

Penne with Grilled Chicken and Pesto

Turkey Meatballs in Tomato Garlic Sauce

Greek-style Meatballs with Rice

Skillet Steak with Mushrooms

Spicy Sautéed Veal Chop

Citrus Glazed Salmon

Lemon Sole with Parsley Sauce

Slimmer Linguine with Shrimp

Slimmer Baked Ziti

Fettuccine with Creamy Yogurt Sauce

Orange Banana Chocolate Crisp

Slimmer Shrimp Salad

Cooked baby shrimp can be found in the freezer section and are perfect for this salad enjoyed at Maria and Eleni's Taverna, although you may also use larger shrimp, roughly chopped, in a pinch.

I 1/2 cups cooked baby shrimp
I scallion, trimmed and sliced
2 Tablespoons nonfat plain Greek yogurt
2 teaspoons low-fat mayonnaise
I teaspoon cocktail sauce
Salt and pepper to taste
I cup lettuce leaves, shredded
2 baby red or yellow potatoes, cooked and sliced
A splash of tarragon vinegar
I teaspoon chopped fresh dill (optional)

1. In a medium-size bowl combine the shrimp, scallion, yogurt, mayo, cocktail sauce, and salt and pepper. Gently stir to combine, and refrigerate until ready to serve.
2. For serving, spread the lettuce on a plate, mound the shrimp salad in the middle, arrange the potatoes around, and add a splash of vinegar and the dill, if using.

Makes 1 serving

Slimmer Potato and Egg Salad

A popular combination all over the globe gets a Greek makeover in this surprisingly rich and creamy version using Greek yogurt. Visitors to the Taverna can't resist Maria and Eleni's version of the dish.

2 medium-size red or yellow potatoes
Salt and pepper to taste
A splash of vinegar
1 teaspoon olive oil
1 large hard-boiled egg, peeled and chopped
1 scallion, trimmed and thinly sliced
2 Tablespoons finely chopped green bell pepper
2 Kalamata olives, chopped and pitted
1 teaspoon chopped fresh dill
2 Tablespoons nonfat plain Greek yogurt
2 teaspoons low-fat mayonnaise
1 teaspoon prepared mustard
1 or 2 Tablespoons low-fat milk, to thin, if desired
Lettuce for serving, shredded

1. Place the potatoes in a small saucepan, add enough cold water to cover and a pinch of salt, and boil until fork tender, about 20 minutes.
2. When potatoes are cool enough to handle but still warm, dice and transfer to a medium bowl. Gently fold in the vinegar and olive oil and refrigerate until cool, about 30 minutes.
3. Add the egg, scallion, bell pepper, olives, and dill, and stir gently. In another bowl stir together the remaining ingredients, adding a bit of milk to thin. Pour over the potato mixture, fold to coat well, and season to taste with salt and pepper. Chill at least 1 hour before serving over a bed of shredded lettuce.

Makes 1 serving

Salmon Salad Platter

A mix of baby lettuces is particularly good as a base for this salad platter. Bring your dressing in a separate container for workday lunch and pour just before serving.

2 cups spring greens or baby lettuces
1 small cucumber, thinly sliced
1 scallion, trimmed and sliced
1 Tablespoon chopped fresh dill
3 Tablespoons low-fat or nonfat cottage cheese, well drained
2 oz smoked salmon slices
1 teaspoon capers, drained and rinsed

For the dressing:
1 teaspoon prepared mustard
Juice of 1/2 a lemon
2 teaspoons olive oil
Salt and pepper to taste

1. Arrange the greens around the edge of a serving dish or in a large airtight container. Place the cucumber slices around and scatter the scallion and dill.
2. Mound the cottage cheese in the middle and drape the salmon slices over it. Sprinkle the capers on top and refrigerate until ready to serve.
3. In a small bowl or container stir together the dressing ingredients and pour just before serving.

Makes 1 serving

Slimmer Salad Platter

This is a delightful presentation and very easy to compose the night before. Try filling your tomato on other occasions with chicken salad, shrimp salad, or cottage cheese.

2 cups mixed lettuce
I medium tomato
1/2 small cucumber, sliced
I scallion, trimmed and sliced
3 green bell pepper circles
A pinch of salt

For the tomato filling:
2 large hard-boiled eggs, peeled and chopped, or
  One 3.5 oz can solid white tuna in water, well drained
2 Tablespoons nonfat plain Greek yogurt
2 teaspoons low-fat mayonnaise
I teaspoon prepared mustard
Fresh ground pepper

Lemon wedge, for serving

1. Arrange the lettuce around the edge of a serving dish or in a large airtight container.
2. Core the tomato and make 6 cuts down from the center almost to the bottom, leaving the tomato intact. Gently fan out like a star shape and shake out any excess liquid. Put in the center of the dish or container.
3. Scatter the cucumber, scallion, and bell pepper around the tomato and add a pinch of salt over all.
4. Make the filling by gently stirring together all the ingredients in a small bowl. Mound in the center of the tomato, cover, and refrigerate until ready to eat. Serve with the lemon wedge.

Makes 1 serving

Marinated Vegetable Salad

**You'll be whisked to the Mediterranean in no time when you taste
this antipasto-type salad that's also full of healthy fiber and nutrition. A delicious first course dish from Maria and Eleni's Taverna that
should be prepared the night before enjoying.**

2 teaspoons olive oil
I small onion, diced
I small celery stalk, diced
I small carrot, diced
I garlic clove, minced
Salt and pepper to taste
I Tablespoon balsamic vinegar
1/2 cup tomato sauce
2/3 cup water
1/2 medium potato, diced
1/2 cup frozen peas, thawed
1/2 cup canned or frozen artichoke hearts without oil, drained
   and roughly chopped
I Tablespoon chopped fresh dill
I oz reduced fat cheese, such as Provolone or mozzarella,
   diced

1. Heat the oil in a large nonstick skillet over medium-high
   heat. Add the onion, celery, and carrot and cook, stirring
   for 2 minutes without browning. Add the garlic, sprinkle
   with salt and pepper, and cook a further minute.
2. Stir in the vinegar, tomato sauce and water, and bring to
   a simmer. Add the potato, peas, and artichokes, and again
   bring to a simmer. Reduce the heat, cover, and cook until
   the vegetables are tender, about 10 minutes.
3. Remove from the heat and stir in the dill. Transfer to a container and allow to refrigerate overnight. Before serving,
   stir in the cheese.

Makes 1 serving

Mediterranean Chickpea Salad

Full of fresh flavor with a hint of spice, not to mention a good amount of healthy fiber, this salad will satisfy any size appetite, just as it has at Maria and Eleni's Taverna for years!

One 15 oz can chickpeas, drained and rinsed
1 scallion, trimmed and thinly sliced
1/2 small cucumber, seeded and diced
2 Tablespoons diced green bell pepper
1 plum tomato, cored, seeded, and diced
2 teaspoons chopped fresh parsley
1 teaspoon capers, drained and rinsed
A dash of cayenne pepper
Juice of 1/2 a lemon
2 teaspoons olive oil
1 teaspoon balsamic vinegar
Salt and pepper to taste
1 teaspoon prepared mustard
A pinch of dried oregano

1. In a medium bowl toss together the chickpeas, scallion, cucumber, bell pepper, tomato, parsley, capers, cayenne pepper, and lemon juice. Set aside.
2. In a small bowl stir together the remaining ingredients and pour over the chickpea mixture. Toss well to coat and allow to marinate, stirring occasionally, for at least 1 hour before serving.

Makes 1 serving

Slimmer Club Sandwich

Less bread but more flavor in this healthy version of a classic lunch. Look for sprouts in the organic produce section of your supermarket.

For the spread:
1 Tablespoon nonfat plain Greek yogurt
1 teaspoon low-fat mayonnaise
1 teaspoon prepared mustard
1 teaspoon ketchup

2 light whole wheat bread slices, toasted
2 oz grilled chicken breast fillet, sliced
1 slice reduced fat cheese, such as Swiss or Munster
3 slices tomato
1/2 cup broccoli or alfalfa sprouts

1. Make the spread by stirring together the ingredients in a small bowl and keeping refrigerated until ready to use.
2. Compose the sandwich by putting half the spread mixture on one side of each slice of toast. Layer the chicken, cheese, tomato, and sprouts on one slice, top with the other, secure with toothpicks, and cut into 4 triangles. Wrap in foil and refrigerate or serve immediately.

Makes 1 serving

Bean and Vegetable Chowder

This soup is a snap to put together and is worth doubling or even tripling the recipe to have on hand for Free Days. It also freezes well.

1 teaspoon olive oil
1/2 small onion, diced
1 small celery stalk, sliced
1 small carrot, sliced
1/2 cup white or Savoy cabbage, shredded
Salt and pepper to taste
1 1/2 cups vegetable or chicken broth
1/4 cup tomato sauce
1/4 teaspoon *each,* dried oregano and basil
1/2 medium potato, diced
1 cup canned red or white kidney beans, drained and rinsed

1. Heat the oil in a medium saucepan over medium heat and add the onion, celery, carrot, and cabbage. Season with salt and pepper and cook, stirring often, until the vegetables are somewhat softened, about 4 minutes.
2. Stir in the broth, tomato sauce, herbs, and potato, and bring to a simmer. Reduce the heat and cook, stirring occasionally, until all the vegetables are tender, about 15 minutes. Stir in the beans and cook another 2 minutes.
3. Taste for seasoning and serve immediately or transfer to a container to refrigerate or freeze.

Makes 1 serving

White Bean Soup

You can also make this from dried beans by soaking them in water overnight, rinsing, and cooking them in fresh water until tender. Then add as indicated in the recipe below.

2 teaspoons olive oil
1/2 small onion, chopped
1/2 medium carrot, diced
1/2 small celery stalk, diced
Salt and pepper to taste
1 cup low-sodium chicken broth
1/2 cup water
One 8 oz can tomato sauce
One 15 oz can cannellini beans, drained and rinsed
A pinch of rubbed sage

1. Heat the oil in a medium saucepan over medium-high heat and add the onion, carrot, and celery. Season with salt and pepper and cook, stirring until the vegetables have softened, about 4 minutes.
2. Add the remaining ingredients, bring to a simmer, reduce the heat to medium-low, and cook for 8 minutes.
3. Using an immersion blender or a potato masher, break down some of the beans to thicken the soup. Taste for seasoning and serve immediately.

Makes 1 serving

Slimmer Sausage Pizza

Italian-style turkey or veal sausages from the butcher would also be delicious here, but you'll want to cook them by grilling or roasting first before slicing and adding as a topping.

1 individual pre-baked pizza crust (for homemade crust,
    see p. 116)
2 Tablespoons marinara sauce (for homemade sauce,
    see p. 114)
3 Tablespoons shredded reduced fat mozzarella
2 Tablespoons shaved onion
4 red or green bell pepper rings
1 medium pre-cooked Italian-style chicken sausage, sliced

1. Preheat the oven according to pizza crust instructions. Place the crust on a baking sheet and spread the sauce over. Sprinkle the cheese over, distribute the onion and bell pepper evenly, and top with the sliced sausage.
2. Bake according to package instructions until the cheese melts and the pizza is well heated and crisp on the edges, about 12 minutes. Remove from the oven and transfer to a serving dish.

Makes 1 serving

Greek-style Phyllo Calzone

Phyllo can be found in the frozen department of your supermarket. Always be sure to keep it well wrapped to avoid drying out.

2 teaspoons olive oil
1/2 small onion, diced
1/4 cup diced green bell pepper
1/4 cup chopped white mushrooms
Salt and pepper to taste
1 medium pre-cooked Italian-style chicken sausage, diced
1/2 cup marinara sauce (for homemade, see p. 114)
2 sheets phyllo, thawed and kept under a damp paper towel
1/2 cup reduced fat mozzarella

1. Heat 1 teaspoon of the olive oil in a medium nonstick pan over medium-high heat. Add the onion, bell pepper, and mushrooms, sprinkle with salt and pepper, and cook, stirring often, until the vegetables are tender and lightly browned, about 3 minutes.
2. Stir in the diced sausage and marinara sauce, cook for 2 minutes more, and set aside. Preheat the oven to 350° F.
3. Carefully unwrap the phyllo and cut the layered sheets into 2 equal rectangles. Place them side by side on a nonstick baking sheet.
4. Spoon the calzone filling on one side of both phyllo rectangles. Evenly distribute the cheese on top and fold over to cover. Press the edges together to form a closed packet and brush the tops with the remaining olive oil.
5. Bake until the phyllo is crisp and lightly browned and the filling is bubbly, 20 to 25 minutes.

Makes 2 servings

Garden Vegetable Omelette

Omelette-making using this method is a real snap and a great idea for a quick dinner or weekend lunch. You can vary the vegetables and cheese according to taste and whatever you may have on hand.

I teaspoon olive oil
1/2 small onion, thinly sliced
1/4 cup green or red bell pepper, cut into small dices
1/2 cup thinly sliced mushrooms
I plum tomato, seeded and diced
Salt and pepper to taste
I large egg
I large egg white
I Tablespoon reduced fat milk
2 Tablespoons shredded reduced fat cheese
I Tablespoon nonfat plain Greek yogurt
I teaspoon chopped fresh parsley

1. Heat the oil in a medium nonstick pan over medium heat. Add the onion, bell pepper, mushrooms and tomato, season with salt and pepper, and cook, stirring often until the vegetables have softened, about 4 minutes.
2. Whisk together the egg, egg white and milk in a small bowl and pour over the vegetable mixture, spreading out evenly with a wooden spoon. Sprinkle the cheese on top, lower the heat, cover, and cook until the egg is set and the cheese is melted, 2 to 3 minutes.
3. Use a spatula to flip over one side of the omelette and transfer to a serving dish. Top with the yogurt and parsley.

Makes 1 serving

Chicken with Orzo

Quick and easy should be the name of this delicious meal that cooks in one baking dish. You can also prepare this with cubed turkey breast or lamb steak.

1/2 medium onion, finely chopped
1 garlic clove, minced
1 cup diced tomatoes
2 teaspoons olive oil
1/2 teaspoon paprika
Salt and pepper to taste
8 oz boneless, skinless chicken breast, cut into 1-inch cubes
1 cup boiling water
1/2 cup dry orzo
2 Tablespoons grated Parmesan cheese

1. Preheat the oven to 350° F.
2. In a medium-size baking dish with a lid, combine the onion, garlic, tomatoes, olive oil, paprika, salt, and pepper. Stir well to combine.
3. Add the chicken pieces, cover, and bake for 30 minutes, occasionally stirring.
4. Add the water and orzo, stir well, cover, and bake a further 30 minutes until the orzo is tender, stirring occasionally. Serve sprinkled with the cheese.

Makes 2 servings

Herb Roasted Chicken with Vegetables

Aromatic herbs flavor tender chicken and delicious vegetables in this easy one-dish meal.

4 sprigs fresh thyme
4 sprigs fresh oregano or marjoram
2 small plum tomatoes, sliced
2 medium skinless split chicken breasts
Salt and pepper to taste
1 medium red or yellow potato, cut into chunks
1 medium zucchini, trimmed and cut into 1-inch pieces
1 small carrot, cut into 1/2-inch pieces
1/2 cup pearl onions
2 teaspoons olive oil
2 teaspoons chopped fresh parsley

1. Preheat the oven to 375° F.
2. Place the herb sprigs in a single layer in the middle of a medium-size casserole. Cover the herbs with the sliced tomatoes and place the chicken breasts, which have been seasoned with salt and pepper, flesh side down on the tomato and herb bed.
3. In a medium bowl combine the potato, zucchini, carrot, onions, and olive oil and stir well to coat. Scatter the mixture around the chicken, season with salt and pepper, and roast in the oven until the vegetables are lightly browned and tender and an instant-read thermometer inserted in the chicken breast reaches 165° F, about 30 minutes. Occasionally stir the vegetables to brown evenly and prevent sticking.
4. To serve, transfer the chicken to a dish, spoon the tomatoes and other vegetables over, and sprinkle with the parsley.

Makes 2 servings

Chicken and Onion Ragout

Sweet caramelized onions highlight this hearty dish that's full of flavor and spice.

2 teaspoons olive oil
I large onion, thinly sliced
Salt and pepper to taste
Two 3 to 4 oz boneless, skinless chicken breasts
I Tablespoon balsamic vinegar
1/2 cup crushed tomatoes
I Tablespoon tomato paste
I cup low-sodium chicken broth or water
I bay leaf
A pinch of ground allspice
A pinch of ground cloves

1. Heat the oil in a large nonstick skillet over medium-high heat. Add the onions, season with salt and pepper, and cook, stirring often until the onions are soft and browned, about 10 minutes.

2. Season the chicken with salt and pepper and add to the skillet, cooking for 2 minutes on each side. Stir in the vinegar and cook until evaporated. Add the remaining ingredients, stir well to combine, bring to a simmer, cover, reduce the heat, and cook until the chicken is firm and no longer pink, about 20 minutes.

3. Remove the chicken from the skillet, discard the bay leaf, and reduce the sauce over medium heat until thick. Pour over the chicken and serve.

Makes 2 servings

Penne with Grilled Chicken and Pesto

Having grilled chicken fillets on hand that can be added to salads and pasta is a great idea for quick meal preparation on weekday nights.

For the pesto:
2 teaspoons olive oil
1 teaspoon pine nuts
1 small garlic clove
1/2 cup fresh basil leaves
1 Tablespoon grated Parmesan cheese

2 oz penne pasta cooked according to package instructions, water reserved
1 cup grilled chicken breast fillet, warmed and diced
Salt and pepper to taste

1. Combine the pesto ingredients in a mini chopper or blender and process until smooth.
2. Add the pesto to the cooked pasta, thinning with a little of the hot pasta water. Stir in the chicken, season to taste with salt and pepper, and serve immediately.

Makes 1 serving

Turkey Meatballs in Tomato Garlic Sauce

A hint of Middle Eastern spice highlights these lean and healthy meatballs that are delicious over couscous or packed into a pita pocket.

2 teaspoons olive oil
1/2 small onion, finely chopped
2 garlic cloves, minced
Salt and pepper to taste
1/4 teaspoon each ground cumin, turmeric, and coriander
A dash *each* of ground cinnamon and cayenne pepper
1 cup crushed tomatoes
1/2 cup water

For the meatballs:
4 oz lean ground turkey
1 Tablespoon flaxseed meal
1 Tablespoon ground oats
Salt and pepper to taste
1 garlic clove, minced
A dash of ground cumin
1 egg white

1. Heat the oil in a nonstick saucepan over medium heat and add the onion and garlic. Season with a little salt and pepper and cook without browning, stirring often, for 2 minutes. Add all the spices and stir a further minute.
2. Pour in the tomatoes and water, bring to simmer, reduce the heat to low, and cook to thicken, for 10 to 12 minutes.
3. Meanwhile, make the meatballs by combining all the ingredients in a medium bowl and mixing well with your hands. Form into walnut-sized balls and drop into the simmering sauce. Keep the sauce and meatballs cooking at a low simmer for 25 minutes, until the meatballs are firm and cooked through, stirring occasionally to prevent sticking.
4. Transfer the meatballs to a serving dish, taste the sauce for additional seasoning, and pour over the meatballs to serve.

Makes 1 serving

Greek-style Meatballs with Rice

Part meatball, part rice ball, you'll love these easy-to-make Greek favorites that are full of flavor. Try making with ground turkey or lamb. Diners at Maria and Eleni's Taverna find them hard to resist!

For the meatballs:
8 oz lean ground beef
Salt and pepper to taste
1/2 cup cooked brown rice
2 Tablespoons flaxseed meal
1 Tablespoon ground oats
1/2 small onion, finely chopped
3 sundried tomato pieces, finely chopped
1 teaspoon each chopped fresh dill, mint, and parsley
1 egg white

2 teaspoons olive oil
2/3 cup water
Juice of 1/2 a lemon
1 teaspoon cornstarch

1. In a medium bowl combine all the ingredients for the meatballs and mix well, using your hands. Shape into walnut-size balls and place on a sheet of wax paper. Set aside.
2. Heat the olive oil in a large nonstick skillet over medium-high heat. Add the meatballs, one at a time, allowing a little space in between each. Cook over medium heat, turning occasionally to brown evenly.
3. Add the water to the skillet, stir, and scrape up any browned bits, cover, reduce the heat to low, and cook until the meatballs are firm and no longer pink inside, 5 to 8 minutes.
4. Remove the cover, stir together the lemon juice and cornstarch, add to the skillet, and swirl the pan to create a light coating of a sauce for the meatballs. Serve immediately.

Makes 2 servings

Skillet Steak with Mushrooms

Flavorful sautéed mushrooms top a quick-cooking lean steak that's perfect when served alongside a crisp green salad.

1 teaspoon olive oil
One 3 to 4 oz beef fillet mignon or boneless sirloin steak
Salt and pepper to taste
A pinch of dried oregano
1 cup sliced white mushrooms
3 Tablespoons dry white wine

1. Heat the oil in a medium nonstick skillet over medium-high heat. Season the steak with salt, pepper, and a little oregano.
2. Sear the steak on both sides until well browned but not cooked through, about 2 minutes per side. Transfer to a plate and set aside.
3. Add the mushrooms to the skillet, sprinkle with salt and pepper, and cook, stirring occasionally, until lightly browned, about 4 minutes.
4. Stir in the wine, return the steak with its juices to the skillet, cover, and reduce the heat to low. Cook to desired doneness, about 4 minutes for medium well. Transfer the steak to a serving dish and top with the mushroom mixture.

Makes 1 serving

Spicy Sautéed Veal Chop

This is a quick and easy method for preparing any type of chop or steak stovetop. You can make the sauce as spicy or as mild as you like!

1 teaspoon olive oil
One 4 to 6 oz veal chop on the bone, trimmed of all fat
Salt and pepper to taste
A dash of dried herbs
2 Tablespoons white wine
1/4 cup low-sodium vegetable broth
1 teaspoon prepared mustard
1 teaspoon ketchup
A dash of Tabasco sauce, or more to taste

1. Heat the oil in a nonstick skillet over medium-high heat. Season the chop with the salt, pepper, and herbs, and brown in the skillet on both sides. Transfer to a plate and set aside.
2. Add the wine to the skillet and cook, scraping up any browned bits from the chop. Whisk in the remaining ingredients, bring to a simmer, return the chop to the skillet with any accumulated juices, cover, reduce the heat to low, and cook the chop until no longer pink inside, 3 to 8 minutes, depending on thickness. Turn the chop periodically to coat with the sauce.
3. Transfer with the sauce to a clean dish and serve immediately.

Makes 1 serving

Citrus Glazed Salmon

The sweet and tangy flavor of citrus fruit is perfect for the salmon in this healthy omega-3 packed dish from Maria and Eleni's Taverna menu that goes straight from fridge to oven or grill.

Two 4 oz salmon fillets, preferably wild caught, skin removed

For the marinade:
Juice of 1 lemon
Juice of 1 orange
1 Tablespoon olive oil
1/4 teaspoon grated orange rind
1 teaspoon prepared mustard
1 Tablespoon chopped fresh dill
Salt and pepper to taste

1. Make the marinade by whisking together all the ingredients in a small bowl.
2. Place the salmon fillets in a ceramic or glass baking dish and pour the marinade over. Cover and refrigerate for at least 2 hours, occasionally turning the fillets.
3. Preheat the oven to 375° F.
4. Remove the cover and bake the salmon in the middle of the oven until firm and pink, about 25 minutes. Occasionally check and move to prevent sticking and to evenly glaze.

Makes 2 servings

Lemon Sole with Parsley Sauce

Light and tangy, this easy fish dinner would go well with steamed vegetables on the side. Feel free to substitute flounder or tilapia in place of the sole.

4 oz fish fillet, such as lemon sole or flounder
Juice of 1/2 a lemon
2 Tablespoons white wine
1 teaspoon olive oil
Salt and pepper to taste
A dash of paprika

For the parsley sauce:
2 Tablespoons nonfat plain Greek yogurt
1 Tablespoon nonfat evaporated milk
1 1/2 Tablespoons finely chopped fresh parsley
1 teaspoon capers, drained, rinsed, and chopped

1. Place the fish fillet in a shallow baking dish in a single layer. Drizzle the lemon, wine, and oil over, and season with the salt and paprika. Add a dash of paprika and marinate in the refrigerator for at least 1 hour.
2. Preheat the oven to 350° F. Meanwhile, whisk together the sauce ingredients in a small bowl and refrigerate until ready to serve.
3. Bake the fish in the casserole dish until firm and white, and the edges begin to brown, about 15 minutes. Transfer to a serving dish and serve with the sauce on the side.

Makes 1 serving

Slimmer Linguine with Shrimp

Keeping a bag of frozen uncooked or cooked shrimp on hand will make this a quick and easy preparation on weekday nights. Try the same method with clams, or a mixed seafood combo. A well-loved meal at Maria and Eleni's Taverna.

1 teaspoon olive oil
1 Tablespoon finely chopped onion
1 garlic clove, minced
Salt and pepper to taste
2 Tablespoons dry red or white wine
1 cup crushed canned tomatoes
1/4 cup water
A dash of cayenne pepper
4 oz medium shrimp, peeled and deveined
2 oz linguine, cooked according to package instructions
1 teaspoon chopped fresh parsley

1. Heat the oil in a medium nonstick skillet over medium heat. Add the onion and garlic, sprinkle with salt and pepper, and cook, stirring, until softened, about 2 minutes. Pour in the wine and cook a further minute.

2. Add the tomatoes, water, and cayenne pepper, bring to a simmer, reduce the heat to low, and cook for 3 minutes, stirring occasionally.

3. Add the shrimp and continue to cook until they are pink and firm, about 2 minutes. Add the linguine, toss to coat, and continue cooking for a minute more until well heated. Serve topped with the parsley.

Makes 1 serving

Slimmer Baked Ziti

You'll love this healthy version of baked pasta that is brimming with nutritious vegetables and the great flavor of roasted garlic chicken sausage.

1 teaspoon olive oil
1/2 small onion, finely chopped
1/4 cup chopped green bell pepper
1/2 cup sliced white mushrooms
Salt and pepper to taste
1 medium pre-cooked roasted garlic chicken sausage, sliced
1 cup prepared marinara sauce (for homemade sauce, see
   p. 114)
1/4 cup water
1 1/2 cups cooked ziti pasta
3 Tablespoons shredded reduced fat mozzarella

1. Preheat the oven to 350° F.
2. Heat the oil in a medium nonstick skillet over medium heat, add the onion and pepper and cook, stirring occasionally, for 2 minutes. Add the mushrooms, season with salt and pepper, and continue to cook until the vegetables are tender, about 5 minutes.
3. Add the sliced sausage, marinara sauce, and water, and bring to a simmer. Cook over low heat for 2 minutes.
4. Remove from the heat and stir in the ziti. Transfer to a medium-size baking dish and top with the mozzarella. Bake until the cheese has melted and the ziti is well heated through and bubbly around the edges, 20 to 25 minutes.

Makes 1 serving

Fettuccine with Creamy Yogurt Sauce

Greek yogurt provides the richness and creaminess without the fat in this amazing pasta dish that is particularly tasty made with spinach fettuccine if available.

2 to 3 oz dry or fresh fettuccine
Salt to taste
1 teaspoon unsalted butter
1 small shallot, finely chopped
1/2 cup nonfat plain Greek yogurt
Freshly ground pepper
1 Tablespoon grated Parmesan cheese

1. Bring a pot of salted water to boil over high heat to cook the fettuccine.
2. Melt the butter in a medium nonstick saucepan over medium heat, add the shallot, sprinkle with salt, and cook until softened, about 2 minutes, being careful not to brown the butter or the shallots. Whisk in the yogurt, remove from the heat, and set aside.
3. Cook the fettuccine according to the package instructions. Transfer with tongs to the saucepan, adding a little of the pasta water to thin the sauce. Stir well to coat, and add the freshly ground pepper. Taste for the addition of salt.
4. Serve immediately, sprinkled with the cheese.

Makes 1 serving

Orange Banana Chocolate Crisp

Rich dark chocolate can turn a simple fruit dessert into a real delicacy! If you can't find chocolate granola, follow the directions below to make your own topping.

1/2 orange, peeled, seeded, and cut into supremes
1/2 banana, peeled and sliced
2 Tablespoons chocolate glazed granola or other wheat cereal

Place the orange and banana in a dessert dish. Top with the granola and microwave for 15 seconds. Serve immediately.

Note: To make your own chocolate topping, sprinkle the granola or other cereal over the fruit and drizzle 1/2 oz dark chocolate that has been melted in the microwave over all.

CYCLE C

Tuna Salad with Citronette Dressing

Lentil Walnut Salad

Slimmer Caesar Salad with Grilled Chicken

Poached Salmon Salad Niçoise

Mediterranean Seafood Salad

Deluxe Garden Salad

Shrimp with Garlic Aioli

Greek Olympiad Pizza

Grilled Chicken Pizza

Whole Wheat Baguette Pizza

Mediterranean Chicken Fricasseé

Chicken with Yogurt Sauce

Summer Vegetable Risotto with Chicken

Turkey Phyllo Pot Pie

Beef and Mushroom Ragout

Florentine Beef Burger

Veal Scallopini with Quick Caper Sauce

Sausage and Peppers with Orzo

Poached Salmon with Root Vegetables

Baked Salmon with Fennel and Tomatoes

Baked Cod Casserole

Greek-style Grilled Fish and Vegetables

Slimmer Pasta Alfredo

Chickpea Curry Stew

Orange Chocolate Crunch Cup

Tuna Salad with Citronette Dressing

Orange and honey highlight this crisp and crunchy salad that's perfect for taking to work. Bring the flaked tuna in a separate container and add just before eating.

1 1/2 cups confetti coleslaw mix (that includes white and red cabbage and carrot)
1 scallion, trimmed and sliced
1 Tablespoon roughly chopped dill sprigs

For the citronette:
Juice of 1/2 an orange
2 teaspoons lemon juice
1 teaspoon mustard
1 teaspoon honey
2 teaspoons olive oil
Salt and pepper to taste

One 3.5 oz can solid white tuna in water, drained and flaked

1. In a medium bowl toss together the slaw mix, scallion, and dill.
2. In a small bowl whisk together the citronette dressing ingredients and pour over the slaw mixture. Toss well to coat, cover, and refrigerate until ready to eat.
3. Serve topped with the flaked tuna.

Makes 1 serving

Lentil Walnut Salad

Walnuts are one of the few nonfish sources of healthy Omega 3 and here they do double duty in this delicious salad that's full of fiber and flavor.

1 1/2 cups cooked brown lentils
1 scallion, trimmed and sliced
1/4 cup diced green bell pepper
2 walnuts, chopped
1 Tablespoon chopped fresh parsley

For the dressing:
1 Tablespoon walnut oil
1 Tablespoon balsamic vinegar
1 garlic clove, minced
1 teaspoon prepared mustard
Salt and pepper to taste

To serve:
Lettuce leaves
1/4 cup cherry or grape tomatoes
A few croutons

1. In a medium bowl gently stir together the lentils, scallion, bell pepper, walnuts, and parsley.
2. In a small bowl whisk together the dressing ingredients and add to the lentil mixture, carefully folding in to coat. Cover and refrigerate for 1 hour or overnight.
3. To serve, arrange the lettuce leaves as a bed, mound the lentils in the middle, arrange the tomatoes around, and top with the croutons.

Makes 1 serving

Slimmer Caesar Salad
with Grilled Chicken

Classic Caesar salad is usually laden with fat but this version is guilt-less and also super delicious. Try adding grilled shrimp in place of the chicken for variety.

For the dressing:
1 small garlic clove, minced
1 teaspoon prepared mustard
1 small anchovy, minced
2 teaspoons olive oil
2 teaspoons low-fat mayonnaise
2 Tablespoons nonfat plain Greek yogurt
Freshly ground pepper

2 cups romaine lettuce
1 slice turkey bacon, cooked crisp and crumbled
2 teaspoons Parmesan cheese, grated
3 oz grilled chicken breast, sliced

1. Whisk together the dressing ingredients in the bottom of a large salad bowl or transfer to an airtight container and refrigerate until ready to serve.
2. Toss the lettuce in the dressing until the leaves are all coated. Add the bacon and cheese, toss again, and top with the chicken.

Makes 1 serving

Poached Salmon Salad Niçoise

You can make the salmon the night before so it is nicely chilled for this salad the following day. If bringing to work for lunch, bring your dressing separately and pour over just before eating.

2 cups mixed lettuces
I plum tomato, quartered
1/2 small cucumber, sliced
1/4 cup French green beans, cooked
I medium red potato, quartered and boiled
  (from the Poached Salmon with Root Vegetables, p. 185)
One 3 to 4 oz poached salmon fillet (from the Poached Salmon
  with Root Vegetables)
4 Niçoise or 2 Kalamata olives
2 small anchovy fillets (optional)

For the dressing:
Juice of 1/2 a lemon
I teaspoon prepared mustard
2 teaspoons olive oil
Salt and pepper to taste

1. In a salad bowl or a large container, toss together the lettuce, tomato, cucumber, green beans, and potato. Break the salmon into bite-size pieces and lay on the top. Sprinkle the olives over and drape the anchovies on top, if using. Cover and refrigerate until ready to serve.
2. Make the dressing in a small bowl or container and pour over the salad just before serving.

Makes 1 serving

Mediterranean Seafood Salad

A variation of the dish served at Maria and Eleni's Taverna. If any of the seafood in the frozen medley is not to your liking you can substitute other ones or simply increase the amount of shrimp.

1 1/2 cups frozen seafood medley (including shrimp, mussels, calamari, and scallops)
1/2 small fennel bulb (stalks removed), trimmed and diced, including some fronds
1 scallion, trimmed and sliced

For the dressing:
Juice of 1/2 a lemon
1 teaspoon mustard
2 teaspoons olive oil
Salt and pepper to taste

To serve:
Mixed greens or arugula

1. Cook the seafood according to the package instructions. Drain and set aside to cool. Add the fennel and scallion and toss to combine.
2. Make the dressing in a small bowl and add to the seafood. Stir well to coat and refrigerate for at least 1 hour or overnight.
3. Serve mounded on a bed of mixed greens or arugula.

Makes 1 serving

Deluxe Garden Salad

This super-sized salad has a variety of crunch and is great for a big appetite. Bring your dressing separately to work and pour over just before serving.

1 cup romaine lettuce
2 cups mixed spring greens
1/4 cup sliced red cabbage
2 Tablespoons shredded carrots
1/4 cup small broccoli florets
1/2 cup cherry or grape tomatoes
1/2 small cucumber, sliced
1/2 small green bell pepper, cored, seeded, and sliced
2 Tablespoons shaved red onion
1 cup chickpeas, cooked
1 hard-boiled egg, sliced
1 oz lean ham, diced

For the dressing:
2 Tablespoons nonfat plain Greek yogurt
2 teaspoons low-fat mayonnaise
1 teaspoon cocktail sauce
A dash of balsamic vinegar
Salt and pepper to taste

1. In a large salad bowl or container combine all the salad ingredients and cover and refrigerate until ready to eat.
2. In a small bowl or container stir together the dressing ingredients and keep refrigerated until ready to serve.

Makes 1 serving

Shrimp with Garlic Aioli

You'll love this dipping sauce which is low in fat but high in flavor and can be used on sandwiches and grilled meats as well.

4 oz large shrimp, cooked, and peeled, tail left on

For the aioli:
2 Tablespoons nonfat plain Greek yogurt
2 teaspoons low-fat mayonnaise
1 garlic clove, minced
2 teaspoons lemon juice
A pinch of salt
A dash of Tabasco sauce

Combine the ingredients for the aioli in a mini blender or chopper and transfer to an airtight container. Refrigerate until ready to use. Serve as a dipping sauce for the shrimp.

Makes 1 serving

Greek Olympiad Pizza

The flavors and ingredients of Greece abound in this winning pizza version that's heads above the rest. You can also use flatbread rounds or oval naan bread for the base.

1 large (12-inch) pocketless pita
2 Tablespoons marinara sauce (for homemade sauce, see p. 114)
1 plum tomato, thinly sliced
1/4 cup thinly sliced red onion
1/4 cup thinly sliced green bell pepper
1 teaspoon olive oil
A pinch of dried oregano
3 Tablespoons crumbled feta cheese
2 Kalamata olives, chopped

1. Preheat the oven to 400° F. Place a baking sheet in the oven while heating.
2. Spread the sauce evenly over the pita, and decoratively place the tomatoes, red onion, and bell pepper on top. Drizzle with the olive oil and sprinkle with the oregano. Top with the cheese and olives.
3. Bake on the preheated baking sheet until the pita is crisp on the bottom and edges and the cheese has begun to melt, 8 to 10 minutes.

Makes 1 serving

Grilled Chicken Pizza

Feel free to add any other vegetables to compliment the toppings for this great version of everyone's favorite.

1 individual pre-baked pizza crust
2 Tablespoons marinara sauce (for homemade sauce, see p. 114)
3 Tablespoons shredded reduced fat mozzarella
1 small plum tomato, sliced
1/2 cup grilled chicken breast, diced
2 Tablespoons diced red onion
2 Tablespoons diced green bell pepper

1. Preheat the oven according to pizza crust directions. Place the crust on a baking sheet and spread the sauce over. Sprinkle the cheese on top and place the tomato slices evenly around. Scatter the remaining ingredients over.
2. Bake until the cheese has melted and the pizza is well heated through and crispy on the edges, about 15 minutes.

Makes 1 serving

Whole Wheat Baguette Pizza

French bread pizza gets a wholesome twist in this easy to make satis-fying dinner that's perfect with a tossed salad.

1/2 small whole wheat baguette, sliced horizontally
2 Tablespoons marinara sauce (for homemade sauce, see p. 114)
2 Tablespoons shredded reduced fat mozzarella
1 plum tomato, seeded and diced
2 white mushrooms, thinly sliced
8 thin slices turkey pepperoni

1. Preheat the oven to 350° F.
2. Place the baguette pieces directly on the oven rack, cut side up and bake just until the cut side is lightly toasted, about 3 minutes. Transfer to a rimmed baking sheet.
3. Top the toasted baguette pieces with the remaining ingredients and bake on the baking sheet until the cheese has melted and the bread is crispy, about 5 minutes.

Makes 1 serving

Mediterranean Chicken Fricasseé

A classic chicken stew with an Aegean twist, this is comfort food at its best, enjoyed by everyone who visits Maria and Eleni's Taverna. If you can't find farro, use soft wheat kernels or barley.

2 teaspoons olive oil
1 medium onion, chopped
1 medium celery stalk, diced
Salt and pepper to taste
8 oz boneless, skinless chicken breast, cubed
2 cups low-sodium chicken broth
1 small tarragon sprig
1/4 cup dry farro kernels
Juice of 1/2 a lemon
1 teaspoon cornstarch

1. Heat the oil in a medium nonstick saucepan over medium-high heat. Add the onion and celery, sprinkle with salt and pepper, and cook, stirring often, until the vegetables are somewhat softened, about 4 minutes.
2. Add the cubed chicken and cook, stirring, for 2 minutes. Pour in the broth, and add the tarragon and farro. Bring to a simmer, reduce the heat to low, and cook, stirring occasionally, until the farro is tender, 12 to 15 minutes.
3. In a small bowl combine lemon juice and cornstarch and add to the stew. Allow to cook at a low simmer while stirring for 3 minutes. Taste for seasoning and serve immediately.

Makes 2 servings

Chicken with Yogurt Sauce

This low-fat version of a Greek classic will definitely become a favorite selection. Enjoy over rice or inside a pita pocket.

2 teaspoons unsalted butter
8 oz chicken tenders, cut into halves
Salt and pepper to taste
1 scallion, trimmed and thinly sliced
3 Tablespoons grated reduced fat Gruyere or Swiss cheese
3 Tablespoons grated Parmesan cheese
1 teaspoon finely chopped fresh mint
1 egg plus 1 egg white, beaten
2 cups nonfat or low-fat plain Greek yogurt at room
   temperature

1. Preheat the oven to 350° F. Coat the bottom and sides of a medium casserole dish with 1 teaspoon of butter and set aside.
2. In a medium nonstick skillet melt the remaining butter over medium heat. Season the chicken pieces with salt and pepper and cook in the butter until no longer pink, but not browned, about 5 minutes. Stir in the scallion and cook a further minute. Transfer the skillet contents to the casserole and spread out evenly.
3. When the chicken has cooled somewhat, sprinkle with the cheeses and mint. In a large bowl, whisk together the beaten eggs, yogurt, salt, and pepper and pour over the chicken mixture.
4. Bake in the oven for 30 minutes until the sauce begins to bubble around the edges. Do not allow to boil. Cool briefly before serving.

Makes 2 servings

Summer Vegetable Risotto with Chicken

Here's an easy and healthy twist on a delicious dish using fluffy basmati rice and pre-cut vegetables.

1 teaspoon unsalted butter
1/2 small onion, finely chopped
Salt and pepper to taste
8 oz boneless, skinless chicken breast, cut into bite-size pieces
2 cups frozen mixed vegetables (that include carrot, peas, corn, red bell pepper), thawed
1 1/2 cups low-sodium chicken broth
2 Tablespoons lemon juice
1 teaspoon cornstarch
2 cups cooked white or brown basmati rice, warmed

1. Melt the butter in a medium saucepan over medium heat. Add the onion, sprinkle with salt and pepper, and cook, stirring, for 1 minute. Add the chicken pieces, season with salt and pepper and cook until no longer pink, stirring often, for about 5 minutes.
2. Stir in the vegetables and add the broth. Bring to a simmer, reduce the heat to low, and cook until the vegetables are tender and the liquid has reduced somewhat, 6 to 8 minutes.
3. In a small bowl combine the lemon juice and cornstarch and add to the vegetable mixture. Bring to a simmer and cook, stirring, for 2 minutes more.
4. Remove from the heat and stir in the rice. Serve immediately.

Makes 2 servings

Turkey Phyllo Pot Pie

Light and flaky Greek pastry holds a rich and creamy low-fat filling of delicious turkey and nutritious vegetables.

I cup reduced fat milk
Salt and pepper to taste
A dash of ground nutmeg
I Tablespoon cold water
2 teaspoons cornstarch
1/2 cup shredded reduced fat cheese, such as Swiss or Fontina
I egg yolk, beaten
I cup cooked turkey breast, diced
1/4 small broccoli florets, steamed to fork tender
1/4 cup small cauliflower florets, steamed to fork tender
I Tablespoon frozen peas, thawed
I teaspoon olive oil
2 sheets phyllo, thawed and kept under a damp paper towel
I teaspoon butter, melted

1. Preheat the oven to 350° F. Have ready two 6-inch diameter pie tins on a rimmed baking sheet.
2. Heat the milk with the salt, pepper, and nutmeg in a medium nonstick saucepan over medium heat to just bubbling. Dissolve the cornstarch in the water and add to the milk, stirring constantly, as the mixture thickens and boils for 2 to 3 minutes. Remove from the heat and stir in the cheese until melted. Slowly add the egg yolk and stir well to combine.
3. Add the turkey, broccoli, cauliflower and peas, stir to coat with the sauce and set aside.
4. Brush the pie tins with the olive oil. Cut each phyllo sheet into 8 pieces and use half the squares to line each pie tin. Spoon the filling evenly into each tin and cover with the remaining phyllo, pinching the edges together to seal. Brush the tops with the melted butter.
5. Bake on the baking sheet until the tops are browned and the edges a bubbly, 12 to 15 minutes. Carefully remove from the oven and serve.

Makes 2 servings

Beef and Mushroom Ragout

Reminiscent of beef stroganoff, this quicker and healthier version of a popular combination will surprise you with its richness and flavor.

2 teaspoons olive oil
8 oz beef filet mignon or sirloin steak, cut into very thin strips
Salt and pepper to taste
I medium onion, diced
I cup sliced white mushrooms
I cup low-sodium beef broth
I cup tomato sauce
2 teaspoons prepared mustard
I cup nonfat plain Greek yogurt

1. Heat 1 teaspoon of the oil in a large nonstick skillet over medium-high heat. Add the sliced beef, season with salt and pepper and cook, stirring often, until lightly browned, about 2 minutes. Transfer with a slotted spoon to a clean plate and set aside.

2. Add the remaining oil to the skillet, add the onion, sprinkle with salt and pepper, and cook over medium heat until softened, about 4 minutes. Add the mushrooms and cook a further 2 minutes.

3. Pour in the broth and tomato sauce and stir in the mustard. Bring to a simmer, reduce the heat to low, and cook for 3 minutes. Slowly whisk in the yogurt without allowing the mixture to boil. Cook over low heat until slightly thickened, stir in the browned beef to heat through, and serve immediately.

Makes 2 servings

Florentine Beef Burger

A favorite of Maria and Eleni's Taverna patron Steven Spielberg, this hearty burger rendition that includes feta cheese and sundried tomatoes is enhanced by spinach, which adds substance and flavor.

2 cups baby spinach leaves, steamed, drained, and chopped
8 oz lean ground beef
Salt and pepper to taste
2 Tablespoons flaxseed meal
I Tablespoon ground oats
I Tablespoon chopped sundried tomatoes
I Tablespoon finely chopped onion
I teaspoon dried Italian herbs
2 Tablespoons crumbled feta cheese
I teaspoon olive oil

1. Combine all the ingredients except the olive oil in a medium bowl with your hands. Shape into two burgers and set aside.
2. Heat a grill or broiler to medium-high and brush the burgers with the oil. Cook until the burgers are firm and well grill marked and the inside is to desired doneness, about 5 minutes per side for medium well.
3. Transfer to a dish and serve immediately.

Makes 2 servings

Veal Scallopini with Quick Caper Sauce

Dinner is served in no time with this fast recipe for a restaurant favorite that's perfectly complemented with a crisp green salad.

2 teaspoons olive oil
3 to 4 oz veal scallop, pounded thin
I teaspoon flour
Salt and pepper to taste
3 Tablespoons white wine
I teaspoon lemon juice
I teaspoon capers, drained and rinsed
2 teaspoons prepared mustard
I teaspoon chopped fresh parsley

1. Heat the oil in a large nonstick skillet over medium-high heat. Dust the veal with the flour and season with salt and pepper.
2. Cook the veal in the oil until no longer pink and lightly browned around the edges, about 2 minutes per side. Transfer to a clean plate.
3. Add the remaining ingredients to the skillet and stir well to combine. Bring just to a simmer and return the veal with its accumulated juices to the pan. Turn the veal several times to coat in the sauce and transfer to a serving dish.

Makes 1 serving

Sausage and Peppers with Orzo

Pre-cooked sausages make this dish a snap but you could also use uncooked Italian style turkey or veal sausage once grilled or roasted.

1 teaspoon olive oil
1/2 medium onion, sliced
1/2 medium green bell pepper, cored, seeded, and sliced
1/2 medium red bell pepper, cored, seeded, and sliced
Salt and pepper to taste
1/2 cup water
1/2 cup tomato sauce
1/4 teaspoon dried oregano
1 1/2 medium pre-cooked roasted garlic chicken sausages, cut
   into bite-size pieces
1/3 cup dry orzo, cooked according to package instructions
1 teaspoon chopped fresh parsley

1. Heat the oil in a medium nonstick skillet over medium-high heat. Add the sliced onion and bell peppers, season with salt and pepper, and cook, stirring occasionally, until somewhat softened and just beginning to brown.
2. Pour in the water and tomato sauce, add the oregano, stir well to combine and bring to a simmer. Add the sausage pieces, cover, reduce the heat to low, and cook until the sausages are well heated through and the vegetables are tender, about 5 minutes.
3. Just before serving, stir in the cooked orzo and top with the chopped parsley.

Makes 1 serving

Poached Salmon with Root Vegetables

This method results in the ultimate moist and tender fish. Use the second portion to make the Poached Salmon Salad Niçoise.

For the poaching liquid:
2 cups water
1/4 cup dry white wine
Juice of 1/2 a lemon
1 bay leaf
1 onion, roughly chopped
4 baby carrots, halved
1/4 cup diced celery root (or celery)
1 small parsnip, sliced
2 medium red potatoes, quartered

Two 3 to 4 oz salmon fillets
Salt and pepper to taste
2 teaspoons olive oil
Dill and parsley sprigs

For the sauce:
2 Tablespoons nonfat plain Greek yogurt
2 teaspoons low-fat mayonnaise
1 teaspoon prepared mustard
1 teaspoon lemon juice
1 teaspoon each fresh chopped dill and parsley

1. In a medium saucepan combine the water, wine, lemon juice, bay leaf, and onion and bring to a boil over medium-high heat. Add the carrots, celery root, parsnip, and potatoes, return to a simmer, reduce the heat and cook until the vegetables are fork tender, about 10 minutes. Using a slotted spoon transfer the vegetables to a bowl and set aside the poaching liquid.

2. Preheat the oven to 350° F. Place the salmon fillets skin side down in the center of a 9 x 9-inch glass or ceramic baking dish. Season with salt and pepper, drizzle the olive oil over, and place the herb sprigs on top.

3. Carefully pour the poaching liquid around the fish and place a piece of wax or parchment paper directly on top of the flesh.

4. Poach in the oven until the fish is firm and cooked through, about 15 minutes.

5. Meanwhile make the sauce by stirring together the ingredients in a small bowl and refrigerating until ready to serve.

6. Remove the fish from the baking dish and serve with some of the root vegetables and the sauce.

Makes 2 servings

Baked Salmon with Fennel and Tomatoes

Cooking fennel brings out its aromatic allure which pairs well with citrus and tomato and provides a delicious bed for baked salmon.

2 teaspoons olive oil
I medium fennel bulb, stalks removed, cored, and thinly sliced
1/2 small onion, sliced
Salt and pepper to taste
I cup tomatoes, crushed
Juice of 1/2 an orange
Juice of 1/2 a lemon
1/2 teaspoon orange rind, grated
I Tablespoon fresh dill, chopped
Two 3 to 4 oz salmon fillets, skinned

1. Preheat the oven to 350° F. Heat the oil in a large nonstick skillet over medium-high heat. Add the fennel and onion, sprinkle with salt and pepper and cook, stirring often, until the fennel is nearly tender and lightly browned, about 5 minutes.

2. Add the tomatoes, orange and lemon juices, and orange rind, bring to a simmer and cook, stirring occasionally, for 5 minutes more. Remove from the heat and stir in the dill. Transfer to a medium baking dish and place the salmon fillets on top.

3. Cover and bake until the salmon is firm and cooked through, 15 to 20 minutes. Serve the salmon with the fennel mixture spooned over.

Makes 2 servings

Baked Cod Casserole

Keeping boiled potatoes in the fridge for adding to casseroles, soups, stews, and salads, can be a big time saver. This recipe takes advantage of that, cooking quickly in the oven in just one baking dish.

2 medium red potatoes, boiled and sliced
Two 3 to 4 oz cod or scrod fillets
Salt and pepper to taste
1 garlic clove, sliced
1/2 cup water
Juice of 1 lemon
2 teaspoons olive oil
1 teaspoon prepared mustard
1 plum tomato, thinly sliced
1/2 cup thinly sliced red, orange, or yellow bell pepper strips
A pinch of mixed dried herbs

1. Preheat the oven to 375° F.
2. Lay the potato slices on the bottom of a medium glass or ceramic baking dish. Place the fish fillets on top and season with salt and pepper. Scatter the sliced garlic.
3. In a small bowl combine the water, lemon juice, olive oil, and mustard and pour into the casserole, distributing well. Layer the tomato slices and pepper strips on top of the fish and potatoes, add a pinch of herbs, and bake until the fish is firm and cooked through, and the vegetables are tender. Serve immediately.

Makes 2 servings

Greek-style Grilled Fish and Vegetables

Grilling brings out the fabulous flavor of fresh fish and vegetables in this delicious and quick dinner that can be whipped up any night of the week.

For the basting sauce:
Juice of 1 lemon
1 Tablespoon olive oil
1 teaspoon chopped fresh oregano
1 teaspoon prepared mustard

4 to 6 oz firm fish fillet such as snapper, sea bass, or swordfish
8 oz asparagus spears, steamed to crisp tender
1 medium zucchini, ends trimmed and sliced into 1/2-inch-thick strips
1 medium onion, such as Vidalia, cut into 1/2-inch thick circles
Salt and pepper to taste

1. Prepare the basting sauce by whisking together the ingredients in a small bowl.
2. Preheat a grill to medium-high and lightly coat with oil. Season the fish and vegetables with salt and pepper.
3. Grill the fish and vegetables, basting with the sauce occasionally, until the fish is firm and cooked through, about 4 minutes per side, and the vegetables are tender and nicely grill marked, about 8 minutes.
4. Transfer all to a clean dish and serve immediately.

Makes 1 serving

Slimmer Pasta Alfredo

This low-fat version can't be beat for rich delicious flavor and creamy texture.

I teaspoon unsalted butter
I small garlic clove, minced
1/2 cup low-fat cottage cheese, well drained
I Tablespoon nonfat plain Greek yogurt
I Tablespoon reduced fat milk
Salt and pepper to taste
A dash of ground nutmeg
2 to 3 oz dry pasta, such as fusilli or bowties, cooked according
   to package instructions, water reserved
I teaspoon grated Parmesan cheese, to serve

1. Melt the butter in a small saucepan over medium heat. Add the garlic and a sprinkle of salt and cook gently without browning for 1 minute. Stir in the cottage cheese, yogurt, and milk and continue to stir over very low heat until just heated through, a minute or two.

2. Transfer the mixture to a blender or mini food processor and puree until smooth. Return to the saucepan, season with salt and pepper and add a dash of nutmeg. Set aside.

3. When the pasta is cooked, drain and add to the cheese sauce along with a tablespoon or two of the pasta water, stirring well to coat. Transfer to a bowl and serve immediately topped with the Parmesan cheese.

Makes 1 serving

Chickpea Curry Stew

If you like hot curry dishes, you can make this as spicy as you want.
You can also substitute a variety of cooked beans like kidney or
white beans for a different version.

2 teaspoons olive oil
1 small onion, diced
1 small carrot, diced
Salt and pepper to taste
1 garlic clove, minced
1 teaspoon fresh ginger, chopped
1 teaspoon curry powder
1/4 teaspoon ground turmeric
1/8 teaspoon cayenne pepper or more to taste
1 cup low-sodium chicken or vegetable broth
1/2 cup crushed tomatoes
1 1/2 cups canned chickpeas, drained and rinsed
2 teaspoons lemon juice
1 teaspoon each chopped fresh cilantro and mint leaves
2 Tablespoons nonfat plain Greek yogurt, to serve

1. Heat the oil in a medium saucepan over medium-high heat and
   add the onion and carrot. Season with salt and pepper and cook,
   stirring occasionally, until somewhat softened, about 3 minutes.
   Add the garlic and ginger and cook, stirring, a further minute.
2. Add the curry powder, turmeric, and cayenne, and stir to
   coat the vegetables. Cook for 1 minute as the fragrance
   rises. Pour in the broth and crushed tomatoes and bring
   to a simmer. Stir in the chickpeas, reduce the heat to medium-low and cook, stirring occasionally, until the stew is
   thickened, about 12 minutes.
3. Taste for the addition of seasoning and just before serving,
   stir in the lemon juice and chopped herbs. Serve with a
   spoonful of yogurt on top.

Makes 1 serving

Orange Chocolate Crunch Cup

Chocolate is on the menu in this terrific snack that will brighten your afternoon!

1 large orange, peeled, and cut into supremes
1/2 oz dark chocolate, melted
2 Tablespoons toasted wheat germ

1. Prepare the orange and arrange the segments in a dessert cup.
2. Stir together the melted chocolate and wheat germ, and drizzle over the oranges. Refrigerate until the chocolate has set, and serve.

Makes 1 serving

Frequently Asked Questions

Q: I am a tea drinker and enjoy a cup of black tea in the morning, such as orange pekoe or English Breakfast. Is this allowed?

A: Yes, you can certainly have regular breakfast tea rather than green or herbal tea. Keep in mind, however, that green tea contains EGCG, a catechin that can help you burn more calories as well as containing higher amounts of antioxidants.

Q: Are only 1% milk and yogurt permitted?

A: Nonfat or 2% fat is also fine. When milk or yogurt is called for you can substitute one for the other as well.

Q: I am lactose intolerant and can't consume all the dairy recommended. Can I still do the diet?

A: As we get older many of us are unable to properly digest the lactose in dairy and experience uncomfortable digestive symptoms such as bloating and diarrhea. By all means, you may substitute soy milk and soy products for the dairy. You may also substitute almond milk or coconut milk and their products, provided they are low fat and unsweetened. Consider purchasing those with added calcium to make up for the switch.

Q: Why do you suggest milk at bedtime?

A: Babies are not the only ones that can benefit from the relaxing effects of milk at bedtime. In fact, a warm glass of milk would be even better. Often when people are dieting, it is the late hours when food cravings might hit, so a soothing nighttime beverage could help you to nod off sooner and avoid the temptation of snacking. Chamomile tea would also be appropriate if you prefer not to drink milk or eat plain yogurt at night. Just be sure not to drink anything caffeinated or containing sugar, which could have the reverse effect and keep you up until the wee hours.

    If you choose not to drink milk at bedtime try to fit it in elsewhere during the day. Remember that calcium can help burn calories and fat.

Q: I have a sensitivity to wheat gluten. Can I substitute gluten-free breads and pastas?

A: By all means, you may select gluten-free breads and pastas, many of which are excellent sources of fiber and quite delicious too. You may also substitute 1/2 cup brown rice for a slice of whole wheat bread on any day.

Q: Is it possible to do the diet as a vegetarian?

A: If you are a vegetarian you can certainly follow the Slimmer program with a few modifications. You will want to be sure you are getting an adequate amount of protein so be sure to include equivalent amounts of soy, beans, and pulses in whatever form you like. Tofu, tempeh, bean and vegetable burgers, and soy yogurt are just a few of the possibilities. If you eat eggs, they can be substituted occasionally for chicken and beef. If you happen to eat fish, as some vegetarians will do, that would be an excellent substitute for the other animal proteins on the menus.

Q: When the menu says "large tossed salad" what do you mean, and what about dressing?

A: The large tossed salad eaten at lunch and dinner should consist of about 1 to 2 cups of lettuce greens of any type and about 1 to 2 cups of combined raw salad vegetables such as tomato, cucumber, bell pepper, onion, scallion, radish, or other types of raw vegetables, such as broccoli florets, if you like. Unless otherwise stated, the dressing should always consist of 1 teaspoon of olive oil and a small amount of lemon juice or vinegar.

Q: I sometimes get tired of eating a tossed salad so often. Is there any equivalent selection I can make for variety?

A: Yes! A few times a week you may substitute 2 cups of steamed vegetables for your tossed salad. They should be selected from the following: broccoli, cauliflower, zucchini, onion, spinach or other greens, cabbage, and asparagus. Small amounts of carrots and peas are okay. And remember to serve them with a teaspoon of olive oil and a bit of lemon juice or vinegar, which is important to the fat-burning Slimmer program. Occasionally you may also substitute a low-fat vegetable soup for your salad as well.

Q: Is there a restriction on salt?

A: Try to use salt sparingly and opt for sea salt or kosher salt over traditional fine-grained iodized salt which usually contains non-caking chemicals that can add an unpleasant taste. Mediterranean sea salt is quite flavorful if you come across it in your specialty food store. In addition, fresh ground pepper from a mill can be used as often as you like.

Q: There's no mention of artificial sweeteners. Are these prohibited?

A: The Slimmer program prefers that you not use any artificial sweeteners except for those in the few diet sodas you are allowed per week. This is because these substitutes have absolutely no nutritional value, and they do not prevent you from craving desserts. If you would like to use sugar in coffee or tea, 1 teaspoon of natural or raw sugar may be counted as a Happy Moment.

Q: Are there any particular reduced-fat cheeses you recommend?

A: Spreadable reduced-fat cream cheese or Laughing Cow wedges are good choices at breakfast. Any reduced-fat sliced cheese is also a good choice such as Swiss, American, or Munster.

Q: When the menu says "fruit salad with yogurt" what exactly do you mean?

A: You can make up your own fruit salad from available seasonal fruit provided it contains two equivalent fruits. For example, 1 apple diced and half a banana sliced would constitute a "fruit salad." You can also mix and match from several different fruits as long as you stick with the equivalent amount. For the yogurt, use no more than 1/2 cup of plain reduced fat or nonfat Greek yogurt, which you can mix in with the fruit or dollop on top. Add a sprinkling of cinnamon as well. Remember, too, that you can add a drizzle of honey or syrup as a Happy Moment if you are yearning for something a little sweeter.

Q: Occasionally you specify eating "red fruits" such as cherries, red grapes, or strawberries. Why are they singled out, and are there other "red fruits" that are good to eat as well?

A: Fruit that is red in color, as well as those that are purple and blue, are particularly good for burning belly fat and providing the body with fiber and antioxidants, and are even cancer-fighting. They are singled out so that you are sure to consume an adequate amount each week. You can also select from blueberries, blackberries, raspberries, pomegranate, cranberries, and red currants.

Q: Is there any way I can increase my rate of weight loss? Can I skip a Free Day?

A: Yes! If you would like to lose a bit faster, on the 7th day of the week, instead of choosing a favorite day's menu or having a Free Day, you can have grilled or broiled fish and steamed broccoli for both lunch and dinner. Some people prefer not to be so strict, but if you are up for it and would like to see quicker results, try this once a week.

Q: What do you recommend when eating out? Is it possible to stick with the Slimmer program?

A: Eating out with friends and family is a pleasure we should enjoy and not avoid. It is entirely possible to adhere to your diet and still dine at restaurants for lunch or dinner. Look for menu selections that are grilled such as chicken, fish, or lean cuts of steak such as sirloin or tenderloin, with no marinades or sauces included. And accompany with a salad or steamed vegetables and the olive oil and lemon dressing. You could even enjoy a small glass of wine with your meal and conclude with a coffee including a bit of raw sugar and milk. These will not disturb the mechanics of Slimmer.

What you must avoid, however, are entrees that are fried, heavy sauces and gravies, excess amounts of bread, pasta, and potatoes, and of course, the dessert menu! Select, if you can, a bowl of fresh fruit salad if others are indulging in dessert so that you can linger as well and enjoy the camaraderie.

Q: I have a very hectic work schedule and may not have had time to prepare the meal the night before to bring for lunch. What can I do?

A: You can easily substitute with half a sandwich and a salad. Use a teaspoon of mustard or low-fat mayonnaise and create a healthy sandwich using 1 slice of whole grain bread, sliced turkey, chicken, smoked salmon, low-fat cheese, or a small can of tuna. If there is no time to cut up your salad to bring with you, visit a local salad bar at lunchtime and fix it there. Keep a small bottle of olive oil and vinegar at work on hand and you will be ready when there is little time to fix and plan.

Q: Sometimes I get home from work and am too hungry and tired to even think about cooking. Can I occasionally have a microwave frozen dinner?

A: Everyone has days when the idea of preparing a meal is just too overwhelming. Rather than take the chance of eating the wrong things, you can certainly keep some healthy frozen entrees on hand in the freezer to serve up quickly a few times a week. When selecting these products, look for those that primarily contain lean protein and vegetables with few carbohydrates such as pasta, potatoes, and rice. Accompany with a salad and a scoop of cottage cheese. You may also, up to twice a week, substitute a canned soup for your meal. Select healthy vegetable- and protein-based varieties, while staying away from cream-based and high-carbohydrate choices.

Q: Can the recipes be doubled or tripled and frozen for the days that I don't feel like cooking?

A: Absolutely. In fact, if you like you can spend a Saturday or Sunday cooking several dishes from the Slimmer recipes and packaging them up into portions and storing them in the freezer for the coming week.

Q: Can I purchase a rotisserie chicken or turkey breast on my way home for dinner with a salad?

A: This would be an excellent approach on a busy night. Be sure to remove the skin before eating and consider using some of the leftovers for lunch in a half sandwich.

Q: Is there any particular exercise recommended on the Slimmer program? Should I join a gym or begin to work with a personal trainer?

A: All dieting can benefit from an exercise program. The more you move, the more you will burn—calorie and fat-wise. Although there is no specific plan recommended, try to incorporate something that you really enjoy, whether it be swimming, walking, or even dancing, so that you will stick with it. Bring a friend along or join a club if that is what will motivate you.

A healthy lifestyle includes some type of exercise on a daily basis and once you begin to lose your excess weight, you will probably feel more like moving about and enjoying the feeling of lightness. It may be difficult at first to adhere to a routine, but don't give up. Do what you can when you can. Eventually it will become a natural part of your life.

Chapter 3

Maintaining Your Success

Congratulations! You've done it! You've reached your ideal weight. In order to maintain that ideal weight, however, you will need to permanently adopt the good diet habits and lifestyle of the Slimmer program.

Every day of Maintenance is actually a Free Day. This means that one of your main meals each day can be a food that you used to enjoy before beginning the Slimmer program, such as a cheeseburger (see page 29 for detailed information on Free Days). The same rules that applied for the Free Days during the cycles, however, apply in Maintenance as well. Shun the fries for a salad and substitute the side order of pasta for vegetables. If in the past, you were eating these favorite foods in large quantities, during Maintenance you will find yourself eating smaller portions (which are really normal portions) but still enjoying the experience. This is because you've learned new dietary habits and are now applying them for life. By working the Slimmer program you have also learned the value of balance and moderation and these tools will be vital to your continued success.

The big difference between previous Free Days and your Maintenance days is the number of Happy Moments you will be allowed as well as the caloric and fat composition of those selections. For example, now you can have two Happy Moments per day and you can have regular ice cream rather than low-fat ice cream. So your selection might be a medium bowl of regular chocolate ice cream. This is perfectly fine. There may even be an occasion when you would like to add a spoonful of hot fudge to your ice cream. This would count as a third Happy Moment and is also fine to enjoy (although not every day!).

However, any more than three Happy Moments per day means that you are in danger of jeopardizing all your hard work and may signal that you are beginning to go off track. It's true, we can all have a bit of a slip now and again. Holidays, hectic schedules, and unexpected life events can wreak havoc on our diets! Just return to the Maintenance rules as soon as possible, and if you need to, skip your Happy Moments one day to accommodate for the previous day's overindulgence.

Whether you realize it or not, you will instinctively know when it is time to take a step back and examine your Maintenance eating. This is because the many weeks of successful Slimmer eating have now become a part of the new you. Make an honest assessment of your current eating habits, but never get discouraged or feel as if you have failed. Simply return to what you have learned and move forward each day with a goal of health and happiness.

Living the Slimmer Life

Remember our island of Crete participants from the Seven Countries Study—the Mediterranean population at that time considered to be the healthiest and longest living people in the Western world? After the survey was complete, the researchers put together a composite description of who this healthy person might be and what his or her life might be like on a daily basis. Here are some of the highlights they found:

· An appreciator of nature and the outdoors, through work and/or pleasure
· An avid walker, to work or on errands
· A social person who knows and greets neighbors and members of the community
· Someone who knows when to relax and find stress-free moments during the day
· A consumer of local fresh fruit and vegetables, with the addition of some lean protein and minimal amounts of alcohol and treats
· A lover of family and friends and the good, simple things in life
· Someone whose life is both fulfilling and rewarding—physically, mentally, emotionally, and spiritually
· Someone like the Slimmer you!

SLIMMER
It's about more than losing weight . . .
It's about how you can become a
better person

PART TWO

THE PSYCHOLOGY OF
SLIMMER

Activating Your Goal:

How to Get to and Maintain Your Ideal Weight

Consider the following 9-point action plan:

1. **ACKNOWLEDGE the pain:** Accept that you're upset, sad, tired, and frustrated with your current weight and health.

2. **Specifically OBSERVE what causes these feelings:** Observe the conditions and situations, and the feelings inside you and around you that contribute to the unhappiness you feel being overweight.

3. **THINK and FEEL about the alternative:** Imagine what it would be like to rid yourself of these excess pounds and unhappy feelings as you strive towards your own ideal weight.

4. **ANALYZE your reasons for losing weight:** Think about why you want to become slimmer (to feel better, to look better), and how your life is negatively impacted by remaining overweight. Repeat these analyses constantly.

5. **CREATE incentives for losing weight:** These are springboards that will give you the drive and power to

stick with your weight-loss plan (a vacation, new outfit, or other reward).

6. **DECIDE to begin:** You've made your decision. Express it constantly and happily. Say to yourself, "I can and will get to my ideal weight."

7. **ACT on your commitment:** Make a daily effort by going on the SLIMMER nutritional program, drinking more water, and increasing your physical activity.

8. **EMPOWER your effort:** Emit positive thoughts and energy for success. Feel good about your effort.

9. **WITNESS the results:** You've now lost all your excess pounds, and have achieved your ideal weight. Remember: To maintain your ideal weight forever, you need to permanently adopt the good dietary habits of the Slimmer program.

Slimmer is a Life Choice

Getting rid of excess pounds may only be a decision that you've made at the beginning, but the reality of shedding those pounds will depend upon your actions and your choices.

Keep in mind that

LIFE IS NOTHING BUT A SERIES OF CHOICES.

Remain devoted to your goal at all times and you will surely succeed. Just about all our life achievements are the result of combining persistence, desire, and focus on what we would like to see happen. This is no different.

And remember to be patient with yourself. Good results come to those who know how to wait and work towards their goals. Believe that you are this type of person and the success of weight loss will be yours.

Making Changes

In order to continue your success and maintain your weight loss, certain changes must occur within yourself. It is important to learn about your own personal triggers that jeopardized your dieting in the past and how specific incidents or feelings may have led you to becoming overweight. Until you are able to face these challenges, you could be destined to repeat the same mistakes over and over and be unable to maintain any weight loss you manage to achieve.

In many ways, the emotional issues and psychological obstacles to weight loss are reflected in our everyday lives in differing contexts. Ironically, if you view your current weight problem as a blessing in disguise, by achieving your weight-loss goals and making significant behavior changes, you could ultimately improve every aspect of your life. Seize this as an opportunity to make the changes you need for a fulfilling and satisfying life on all levels.

A New Relationship with Food

Throughout our lives all of us face difficulties and problems. The problem you face today, as you embark on this weight-loss program, is the unhealthy relationship with food that has become a part of your daily life. By admitting that you alone are responsible for this—through poor nutritional habits, overeating, and lack of physical activity—you can begin a better relationship now. Forgive yourself but also congratulate yourself for now facing up to the realities of your relationship with food. Vow to create a solid, healthy, and beneficial relationship that will help you achieve your ideal weight and improve your life.

How do you do this?

First of all, you must stop thinking and acting as you did before in regard to your relationship with food, because this type of thinking and behavior created the conditions in your life today. Your overweight self has probably been characterized by an obsession about anything that has to do with food—maybe rich desserts are your downfall. Moderation has most likely not been an option. And, as a result, you have been dependent, dominated, and perhaps even enslaved by food—it has been in control, not you. Depression, frustration, and pain have been common feelings.

But this pain and the psychological pressure you have felt have been the wake-up call that has told you to become more moderate (reasonable portions of food; a small daily dessert) and finally acquire a sense of balance. You need to replace your old, bad dietary habits with the new, good habits established in the Slimmer program (for example, instead of eating a chocolate pastry, trying the Banana with Chocolate in the Happy Moments section). If you ignore the wake-up call and the message to change, you will simply spiral into a deeper and more painful state.

However, know that once you understand the lesson you need to learn and then begin to act on it, there will come a day when you will be grateful for having experienced this time, as it helped you change your life by teaching you moderation—a proper portion of everything—and also helped you and your family adopt a good, healthy diet.

Change Takes Time

Your negative thoughts and actions over the years have brought you where you are today: with excess pounds. You certainly did not go to sleep one night and wake up 60 pounds heavier! People who put on weight do not reach this point from one isolated moment to another; every eating splurge is added on to the previous one, and the result is that you gained two pounds in one month, four the next, and finally became overweight.

These facts of the past cannot change, but now you can change this direction toward the positive with patience and dedication to your goal of establishing healthy dietary habits, which will soon become a normal way of life.

It is, therefore, your decision to get rid of your excess pounds and get to your own ideal weight by adopting the good nutritional habits in the Slimmer program, eating reasonable quantities of food, and increasing your physical activity.

YOU CAN LOSE WEIGHT BECAUSE YOU SIMPLY BELIEVE YOU CAN!

Appeal to Your Better Self

Sometimes our ego, the selfish and immature side of us, gets the upper hand and becomes dominant in our lives, taking control over what we know is a better, higher self and way of thinking. When we're overweight, the ego can cause unhappiness through internal ridicule and criticism: *I am not thin enough,* your ego convinces you, *like models or actors.* Eventually we begin to believe—consciously or subconsciously—we are not good enough or worthy enough for a happy life until we are thinner!

And so, we go on extremely restrictive diets to stop the ridicule and pain. Short successes are followed by relapses and more ridicule. We begin to eat poorly again and put on even more weight. The cycle never ends and we are perpetually dissatisfied with our lives and our weight.

Sometimes it is necessary to reach this bottom level of hopelessness and anxiety before we are able to move forward. (This is true not only for poor dieting habits but also for many other addictions.) But once we are able to realize that there is no way but up, a part of our better selves—the mature part—helps us to pick up the pieces and begin a new and better way.

How You Became Overweight . . . and How You Can Deal with It

Consider the following scenario:

1. Perhaps you don't like your life. Negative conditions that are part of your daily existence, such as your love life, work, or family have made you feel unhappy. After a period of time, the unhappiness may turn to distinct sadness, anxiety, bitterness, and anger. Now accustomed to thinking negatively, you feel that you are incapable of success or feel you are worth nothing. You grow angry even at yourself (the ego at work).

2. Because of your inflexible and uncontrollable ego, you turn your anger toward yourself and wonder why you have allowed this to happen to you. Why on earth is everything in your life turning out badly? And perhaps, since you have never been taught to adapt and learn from your mistakes or bad circumstances, you choose to punish even yourself.

3. The price of the anger you inflict upon yourself by punishing yourself "conveniently" (uncontrolled eating of food, desserts, alcohol) turns out to be unwanted weight gain, obesity, and a tendency toward depression. "You only deserve to eat!" This is what you always said to yourself.

4. Now, seeing the price you have paid with your own body (the excess weight) and the great pain or frustration you are feeling in your life, you may now be able to finally start making the change—gradually adjusting to acceptance of your situation and awareness that you can indeed do something about it. Be sure to observe the emotion that results

from the "negative" event—a failed relationship, for example, or family problems—and what vulnerable point in your psyche it corresponds to—that is, why it gets you down. Then work on your own psychological weakness: observe it, acknowledge it, accept it, and analyze it. By doing so, you will be able to understand how it came about and then how it manifested itself in you. You'll learn about yourself, how you were, and, from a new source (Slimmer psychology), how to overcome these conditions. By changing your reaction to what hurts you, you take away its power to cause pain. You will no longer be the same!

Remember:

**DISPLEASURE + INFLEXIBLE EGO
= SADNESS, ANXIETY, BITTERNESS, ANGER**

**ANGER + POWERFUL, UNCONTROLLABLE "EGO"
= OBESITY**

**OBESITY + SEVERE PAIN + FAILED, DEPRIVING DIETS + EVEN GREATER PAIN
= NEED FOR A BETTER AND MORE MATURE SOLUTION**

**NEED + KNOWLEDGE FROM SLIMMER
= THE START TO CREATING A NEW,
SUPERIOR MIND AND BODY**

Why You Did Not Manage to Lose Weight in the Past

Despite numerous attempts at losing weight in the past, you have not been able to shed the pounds and keep them off long term. You dealt with the *result*—that is, your obesity—by trying to magically make your excess pounds disappear with restrictive diets, magical pills, or even surgeries, but you did not deal with the *cause*.

Specifically, you did not act and involve yourself in the weight-loss process by critically considering the following important aspects of weight control:

1. Your poor dietary habits;
2. Your consumption of large quantities of food, desserts, or alcohol that you turned to because of your negative attitude and your poor psychological state;
3. Your lack of physical activity.

Note: Your poor psychological state was due to your inability to deal with frustration (from ordinary daily things to the most important areas of your life), by seeing it as rejection—this in turn caused great pain.

In order to be in the best possible psychological condition, you must learn to handle some frustration by turning it into a learning experience for yourself that aims at self-improvement. You must deal with the causes of your weight gain so that you are able to opt for different choices:

1. Good, healthy dietary habits;
2. Consumption of reasonable quantities of food, desserts, or alcohol; and adoption of a new, positive way of thinking; and
3. Increased physical activity.

More Reasons You Did Not Manage to Lose Weight in the Past

Simply put: *negativity!* Your excess weight is the result of your old, negative way of thinking. In the past, your thoughts went something like this: "Diets are depriving, difficult, and tasteless. I really enjoy food like desserts and other treats. I could never totally withstand these temptations. Therefore, I'll stay overweight forever, since I've never managed to lose weight and keep it off."

By repeating these negative thoughts, you produced emotions of weakness; you "fed" off these emotions and began to feel that you were really unable to follow the rules of good, healthy nutrition. Then you *acted* upon these emotions by behaving in a corresponding way: you continued to eat large quantities of food and desserts because you've convinced yourself that you will never manage to lose weight. In this way, you confirm your initial thoughts and create a self-fulfilling prophecy.

This is why it is necessary to change your thinking. Choose to replace your negative thoughts with positive, more mature thoughts. This means that in order to see only the good side of things and concentrate only on pleasant things, you must begin gathering new, positive information and ideas with which you will systematically and repeatedly feed your mind.

To encourage positive visualization, keep telling yourself, "By splurging in the past, I gained excess weight. From this moment on, however, I am beginning the SLIMMER nutritional program, which includes delicious recipes and Happy Moments. By following Slimmer, I am gradually getting rid of the excess pounds and getting to my ideal weight."

Tune your thoughts in to SLIMMER, and then you'll experience the reality you always wanted: to be healthy and slim.

Positive visualization helped Katie, a 59-year-old office worker, lose 40 pounds on Slimmer. She saw herself eating unnecessarily large quantities of food while imagining the many children of the world requiring sustenance. It literally changed her life and her eating habits forever.

Another reason you weren't able to lose weight in the past is that your effort to fight and be victorious against your dependence on food and desserts was a mistake. You declared war against the foods that you thought caused your weight gain, but in the long run this resulted in you eating even larger quantities of these foods! Very simply put, when your thoughts and acts are aggressive and there is a desire to terminate your bad dietary habits (such as excessive chocolate eating), the part of you that is being attacked almost always reacts by pulling in the opposite direction with very great force.

This kind of action-reaction finally weakens you, because although you use your weapons (eating no chocolate, with statements like, "I'll never eat chocolate again in my life") your dependence recruits its own forces (an irresistible desire to eat chocolate). And your body is, of course, the field of battle in which the war is taking place.

In essence, the more you try to wage war against your dependence on food, desserts, or alcohol, the more their influence over you increases. To get rid of the dependence, you must first of all get rid of any aggression. Do not fight your dependent nature. You must not fight against your bad dietary habits, but rather, you must create new habits that are better and healthier.

Finding Self-Discipline

Many of us struggle with self-discipline whether it be in connection with dieting, working, exercising, or any other aspect of our lives that tends toward extremes. In order to develop this important trait, we need to become aware of our value and respect ourselves. Your body is the temple of your soul, and that is why you must take care of it and not transform it into a garbage basket by eating processed, chemically altered, or plastic food. Say to yourself, "I choose to eat something else and feel proud of my decision."

Get results by setting accessible and realistic goals. Initially you will have small positive results upon which you can stand as a foundation so that you can progress further. The small victories will always lead to bigger ones. Begin by aiming to lose 10 pounds, and later another 10. Don't make your first goal losing 60 pounds. It's too stressful a thought and will hold you back. Reward yourself with emotionally positive actions (you feel great looking in the mirror) and material rewards (small presents to yourself for losing 10 pounds), even for short-term goals.

Control your emotions. Do not allow yourself to get stressed out and upset about your excess pounds any longer. Stop wasting so much energy feeding the negative emotion of repulsion toward your obese self and trying to look like someone else, because that makes you weaker and traps you in the same situation. Your thoughts and feelings, however, can change by changing your beliefs. The new belief should be: Everyone is different, unique. All of your qualities, both internal and external, express your uniqueness and individuality. Accept and praise yourself for what you are today! After all, everything good in your life begins from the moment that you begin accepting your true self, understanding yourself, respecting yourself, and then loving yourself.

Do not regret your past. Accept it as a great teacher in your personal evolution. Stop wasting the present by feeling upset over everything you should or should not have done; you must live only for today and always look forward. This is why you should accept what you look like today and try to adapt positively to the conditions as they exist today. Feel good now, even with your excess pounds.

Techniques to Fend off Negative Thoughts

In your effort to get to your own ideal weight, when a negative thought comes to your mind—for example, a food temptation, such as a slice of cake—don't let it linger. Forget it and replace it immediately with some other encouraging thought (for example, imagining that you've already reached your goal of your own ideal weight).

Begin forming in your mind a picture of yourself without the excess pounds. Envision yourself as slim—how you would feel and act, full of vitality and energy. Focus on what you can actually do with the energy that the proper, healthy Slimmer nutritional program and increased activity have provided you with. Insist on these visualizations, because the human brain functions with images and is radically influenced by them. For even better results, combine the practice of positive visualization with filling your mind with suitable words. Words give substance to power; to access this power when you are faced with a food temptation, begin to repeat:

"My mind NO LONGER CHOOSES to yearn for these things. AS LONG AS I CAN CHOOSE, I choose my own healthy HAPPY MOMENT."

With these techniques, you banish the negative thoughts that inhibit your effort to lose weight, and at the same time exercise your willpower. And it is the power of your will that allows you to make a reality of what you said you would do at the moment that you said it;

that is, to begin the process of ridding yourself of your excess pounds at the present moment. The very fact that you have this desire means that you have the power to make it a reality.

Zoe, a 38-year-old restaurant manager who lost 50 pounds on the Slimmer program, found this method of "changing her thinking" to be instrumental in reaching her weight goals. "I simply kept an image of a slimmer me in mind every time I was tempted."

Public Commitment

Public commitment will help you achieve your own ideal weight. Tell anyone you regularly interact with that you have decided to rid yourself of your excess pounds by faithfully following the Slimmer nutritional program. From the moment that you tell others of your intention, you immediately begin to receive positive pressure to succeed in your goal. Those around you can also provide accountability, support, and cheerleading.

Enjoy the Process

The process of losing weight with the Slimmer nutritional program should be enjoyable, not a depressing chore. Enjoy losing weight. Enjoy eating healthy, delicious food. Learn to relish the unique moments the Slimmer program offers you every day, because you must live and experience today to the limit. Never postpone anything in life! Live in the day, because you will never have it again. Take as much happiness and joy as you can from the journey you are taking to lose weight—do not wait until you reach your destination to feel good. Focus on the recipes in the Slimmer nutritional program that are more to your taste, and do any sort of exercise you wish. Don't do something simply because you should; the only incentive you have to do something is to want it truly, to love it, and to believe that you will derive a lot of benefits from it.

Learn About Basic Nutrition

Everyone can benefit from a little nutritional knowledge. Take the time to read up on protein, carbohydrates, and fats, and you may be surprised at what you learn. For example, fatty acids are created during the production of hydrogenated oil, an ingredient you often find on food packaging, particularly all those very tempting goodies on the cookie shelf. It was developed to stay solid at room temperature and extend the shelf life of manufactured foods. Widely used by local bakeries and the food industry, it is found mainly in desserts, cakes, cookies, crackers, and sausages, and generally in all processed foods and the fried food from fast-food outlets (such as chicken and French fries). Unfortunately, it increases cholesterol levels in the blood, blocks your arteries, and greatly increases the risk of cardiovascular disease, just as saturated fat can do. Avoid these fats, whenever you can, because of the catastrophic effect they can have on your health.

Try this visualization:

Place a small dessert on a plate. Sit in a comfortable armchair, in a quiet place where nothing will interrupt you. Cut off a small piece of the dessert and put it in your mouth. Let it melt, and feel the flavor. Do it again, and concentrate on the fats it contains. Feel the fat it leaves on your tongue. Visualize it mixing in with your saliva and going through your esophagus to your stomach, where the gastric juices turn it into a liquid that, after going to all your vital organs, ends up in the small intestine. There, through your veins, most of the trans fats are absorbed and circulate through your blood in your veins and arteries to your heart.

Now put the palms of your hands together and place your hands on your heart. Try to feel its pulse. Unfortunately, if you have been eating large amounts of food like this for a long time, you may already have fatty deposits like a viscous glue in the arteries of your heart. This is what gradually blocks the flow of blood and leads to a heart attack or stroke. Your heart is now in danger, yet it is what keeps you alive. The only thing it asks of you is to protect it by eating and living in a healthy manner. Don't convince yourself that eating poorly today won't harm you in the long run.

From now on, you have decided to take care of your heart, putting an end to the consumption of food that contains trans fatty acids. Every time you eat something that contains them, try putting a Band-Aid where your heart is so that you remember that you've harmed it!

Cut another piece of the dessert now and put it in your mouth. Don't swallow it; just think of what you've learned about trans fatty acids. Spit it out and throw the rest of the dessert into the garbage. That's where it belongs because of the trans fatty acids it contains. From now on, you will make the right choice of desserts and portion sizes that you've learned about in the Slimmer nutritional program.

By following the Slimmer program, John, aged 27, lost 70 pounds because he learned the importance of eating homemade, delicious food with fresh ingredients, and vowed to never again eat unhealthy processed foods that contain destructive trans fats.

Think what you used to feel when you ate too much, just before you put the first morsel in your mouth. What did you feel? Nervousness, anger, guilt, frustration, sadness, disappointment, loneliness, lack of love, emptiness . . . First of all, accept the main emotion you felt and try to feel it again now. Analyze it very well. Then, go deeper and ask yourself what caused this emotion, and what was not going well in your life. Perhaps it was a lack of communication with your partner; possibly you had problems at work or with your family, or financial difficulties, or even boredom due to loneliness. People turn to addictive behaviors when they do not like what they are feeling and, in order to avoid those unpleasant emotions, they seek an experience that will change their mood, even if it's only temporarily. After all, food, just like alcohol, can create a pleasant mood change, and that is what makes it addictive.

In the past, instead of experiencing and processing your negative emotions, you resorted to eating too much, by eating and swallowing those emotions. All addictive behaviors are efforts to suppress and avoid unpleasant emotions. And, as long as you continue to refuse to deal with your emotions, you prolong the situations that cause them.

Having lost the satisfaction and the feeling of completeness brought about by communicating well with others, having lost love and/or success, you tried to replace them with something else—that is, by eating too much food and too many desserts. This is the madness of addiction, because although food's natural role in life is to nourish us, within an addiction it acquires yet another function: covering emotional needs. The result was that you found yourself in a vicious circle, repeating the same behavior—focused on satisfying your sense of taste—which led you to an even lower emotional level and to a constant gaining of weight.

To stop this sort of addictive behavior, you must work hard with yourself, beginning with an inner process that aims to liberate you from negative emotions. You must not keep those emotions inside yourself. They become suppressed; they poison your soul and manifest themselves as depression and ultimately excess pounds. You must experience your emotions, live through them.

How do you do this? You let them rise to the surface; you allow them to come out, you recognize them, accept them, and then you try to express whatever you feel in words, honestly and precisely. In this way, you will feel relief; you will cease stewing over the same negative thoughts and suffering. When you manage to externalize your negative emotions, they gradually lose their intensity. As soon as they are liberated and you begin to rid yourself of them, they can begin to turn into positive energy, and become tools for change in your personal development.

Learn a new way of life, which besides rejuvenating you will also promote the formation of new, healthy relationships with other people. In healthy relationships, you behave with respect and care towards others. You do not impose your will on them, neither do you control them; you accept them exactly the way they are, without constantly exerting yourself to change them. But be careful: this does *not* mean you should insist on maintaining problematic relationships which you have repeatedly tried to change without getting any results.

Whenever you begin to experience very intense negative emotions that you cannot deal with effectively, try taking concrete action. For example, take a walk, or have a hot, relaxing bath. Teach yourself to associate the negative emotions with another outlet. If you resort to food again, at least make sure that your choices are the lowest in calories, such as a cup of hot, low-fat milk with a level teaspoon of honey, or a small piece of dark chocolate.

Negative feelings about herself crippled Sophia, a 37-year-old business-woman. She realized these thoughts were ultimately manifesting as excess weight when she looked in the mirror. By learning to properly deal with her negative emotions, she lost 65 pounds on the Slimmer program.

Adopt a New, Empowering Philosophy to Deal with Life and Its Problems

There is no doubt that, in order to deal with life and its problems, all of us have adopted a philosophy, a system of beliefs, which defines the manner in which we react to life events. Unfortunately, many people have been trained to believe that they are victims, to mourn over their problems and to constantly curse their "bad luck," while comparing themselves to other people who seemingly have no problems.

By facing life and its problems with this philosophy, you cause yourself constant pain, stress, and sadness. And this may be why you have chosen an addictive relationship with food, desserts, and alcohol—to ease this pain. This addiction is an easy, quick way to avoid experiencing the pain so intensely; it is a temporary escape. If you begin from this moment to face life with a new, empowering philosophy that will get rid of the pain and frustration, then your addiction could end forever.

This strong, new philosophy based on universal truths that will empower you and support you during difficult moments is the following: "You are an inseparable, inextricable part of the Universe. You are a divine creation, a miracle that appeared here as a human being at exactly the moment you were meant to be here. The Universe is perfect and therefore allows nothing imperfect to occur— that is, it does not allow anything bad to happen to itself. Because you, too, are a part of the Universe, whatever happens to you is surely good and beneficial, and will prove in the end to be to your benefit. Therefore, everything occurs in the exact way it had to occur, even if you may not understand it as it happens."

You can conclude from this that you have two basic ways of dealing with your problems: you can either consider them good for you—that is, opportunities for learning—or you can consider them bad. If you choose to think they are good for you, you will be liberated, you will gain hope and optimism, and you will enjoy the steadfast rewards of serenity, success, and a fuller, richer life.

Realize and share with the other people in your life that your happiness does not depend on one thing, or on one person.

Once you adopt this new philosophy, you will avoid the pain from the negative situations in which you were trapped, and you will no longer need substitutes such as food, desserts, or alcohol. To fully become initiated in to this new, empowering philosophy, you must begin to apply it in stages, beginning with the little problems and then expanding to the bigger ones, with your final goal being to adopt it as a stance towards life.

Realize This . . .

Love is a miraculous cure that can help solve your problems. Whatever the problem—such as the obesity you are facing—love for yourself will find a solution for you. And this is why when you understand, accept, and truly love yourself exactly the way you are, it is much more difficult to feel hurt again, regardless of what others may think or say.

In order to take advantage of the beneficial effects of love, you must choose to act only with love. Put love in your every thought, every word, every action. Do not forget that love is a choice that is always inside you. Make that choice now! Always repeat:

EVERYTHING IS LOVE,
and I DESERVE to receive love, as I give
only love to myself and to others.

And Remember . . .

To be successful in your attempt to get to your own ideal weight, read these Slimmer psychology texts *every day.* You must make this a habit, which is why you must do it every day, at the same time, in the same way, and in the same place (if you are traveling, pick a place where you will do it every day in the location where you are staying).

After you begin studying the Slimmer psychology texts every day, they will soon become a part of your conscious mind, but the most important thing is that they will filter through to the unconscious part, the one that gathers all facts, thoughts, and experiences, and which many times makes you act in ways you do not understand, or act without having to think about it beforehand.

And once you've absorbed the meaning of these texts, you will gradually begin to react in a different way to the temptations you face. Soon, with daily practice, the temptations will lessen and following your nutrition plan will become natural. Before you know it, foods and treats that once had power over you will become unappealing. Maintaining your own ideal weight will be as easy as breathing.

Make a solemn vow to yourself that you will never, ever stop the daily ritual of reading the Slimmer psychology texts that aim to support you psychologically and encourage you. There is enormous power in this ritual: use it.

Ellie, aged 63, finally learned to accept and love herself by affirming the Slimmer texts and lost 110 pounds.

MAINTENANCE =
EVERY DAY IS FREE DAY

Now that you are in the maintenance stage, all of your days are Free Days. For this reason, it is extremely important for you to understand the concept of the Free Day. During maintenance you eat healthy food, choosing recipes from the Slimmer nutritional program, but you can also eat what you liked in the past when you were overweight. The difference is that you now eat these foods in reasonable quantities. In other words, you can enjoy your favorite "old" foods, but in ordinary, reasonable portions.

For instance, in the maintenance stage, every day for lunch you can have a moderate portion of your favorite food, without the accompaniments, but you must follow the breakfast, in-between snack, afternoon snack, and dinner of one day of the Slimmer program. You can also enjoy two Happy Moments. This is a Free Day. During maintenance, your Happy Moments can have more calories—you can choose desserts that are not diet desserts.

But remember: a bite-size sweet = 1 Happy Moment; a medium dessert = 2 Happy Moments. An unbreakable rule for Happy Moments is to never, ever exceed 3 Happy Moments daily (the 2 that you are allowed ordinarily, and 1 as a permissible infringement). If this does happen, you lose your Happy Moments for the next day.

How can Happy Moments help you maintain your own ideal weight long term? When you follow the program and deny yourself a treat, you are not doing this to punish yourself, but to enjoy your Happy Moment even more. For example, someone offers you a piece of cake and you don't eat it because you had already planned to have a medium portion of your favorite dessert. You find the strength to refuse the cake because you know that you will enjoy something else that is of greater value to you.

During maintenance, you eat with a different mindset, having acquired a sense of balance; you have finally achieved moderation.

What to Do If You Break the Program

1. **If you break the program only on one day (for example, you went out one evening and overate):** It is possible that someday you may give in to many collected temptations at an event, and exceed your daily maximum of 3 Happy Moments (2 + 1). In this case, on the next day you must restrain yourself and do something to balance the situation. Follow any day of the Slimmer nutrition program, but with no Happy Moments. Try to balance out your nutrition on a weekly basis.

2. **If you break the program for a period of time (Christmas holidays, vacation):** If you go through a period when you break the program and lose your moderation, you must find it again very soon. Your dietary balance is in your hands, and as you've lost it temporarily, you must do something to regain it. Follow any one or two weeks of any cycle of the Slimmer nutritional program.

Remember that you're human: at some point you may become sidetracked. But you must immediately get back to the Slimmer program. You must also keep in mind that by occasionally indulging yourself with too much food, you have not blown all your hard work. You have not destroyed your program, which is proper nutrition with the right, healthy choices.

Remember: When it comes to food, no one is ever perfect. You cannot be perfect everywhere and all the time. Just try the best you can.

In fact, keep this important message in mind:

Lapses are okay
That is, one big dietary splurge is
occasionally all right.
But Backsliding is NOT okay
That is, a string of dietary splurges
is a problem.

For example: You are in the maintenance stage. In a moment of weakness, you succumb to the temptation of eating a large slice of cake. You must put a stop to it there, and not think that because you've broken the maintenance program, you've blown everything sky-high and then continue to eat another large slice of cake, and then a whole pizza, a quart-size soft drink, and then . . . and then . . .

Don't let a lapse—a small slip—become a serious backslide.

A capable and successful person is not one who has never made a slip—in this case, the person who had a big splurge in their diet! A capable and successful person is one who slips up, but then gets up and continues on his path: the path of good nutritional habits. The Slimmer path!

Economize on Calories

Treat the calories you are entitled to every day as something precious. Take care to manage them properly, and avoid being a spendthrift with them.

For example:

A. In a restaurant, avoid eating bread with your accompaniments or starter, and order something that you like, requesting that it is cooked without too much fat, as well as accompanying your meal with a salad of your choice with just a very little bit of dressing on the side.

B. After your meal, share dessert with your friends, and feel empowered because you are satisfied and have eaten less dessert. In fact, by learning to share something that you really love—such as desserts—you gain self-discipline, and you become more giving and generous. You improve and develop as a person; you learn—by offering things—not to be dependent on material things.

When you are in maintenance, you must do the best you can. For example:

A. If you are in a fast-food restaurant, choose your favorite hamburger (without other accompaniments) and drink bottled water or, if you simply cannot resist them, a small portion of French fries and a small diet soft drink. But you must not order a dessert.

B. At an ice cream parlor, if you choose an ice cream for your Happy Moment, make sure that it is a small quantity, and if it's accompanied by whipped cream, do not eat it. If you simply cannot resist it, just try a teaspoonful. The taste alone—not the quantity—will satisfy you.

Now that you are in maintenance, here's a very clever trick. If you have already used the two Happy Moments you are entitled to on a daily basis, and you want to eat something else, you can simply try it! By saying "simply try it" (for example a new flavor of ice cream), it means one, or at most, two level teaspoons, and no more than two separate "trials" a day.

How to Develop a Sense of Portion Size

Make even your most ordinary meal a fancy one, so that smaller portions of food become more important. Eat at a table that has been set properly, so that you can dine without distractions, using ordinary-size porcelain plates, crystal glasses, cutlery, and nice napkins. All of this will lend a formality to your meal, and you will now treat it as a serious activity.

Do not put your whole meal onto one plate. Use at least three plates: one for your salad, one for your accompaniments, and one for the main dish. Serve your food in the center of the plate. Pasta which has been placed tastefully in the center of a pretty plate is definitely more enjoyable to your senses than the same portion that is served untidily.

Eat slowly and chew well; in this way, you improve your digestive processes and enjoy the food more. The faster you eat, the more food you think you need.

If you follow this procedure on a daily basis in your meals, you will manage to create a sophisticated and elegant atmosphere that will inhibit careless, uncontrolled consumption of too much food.

The Importance of Good Quality Ingredients

Take care that your daily menu is based on seasonal, fresh ingredients of the best quality. The secret of the best chefs in the world is using the best ingredients! Schedule weekly shopping trips for the best quality of the ingredients you need to make your meals. Under no circumstances and for no reason must you buy and bring into your home unsuitable and fattening foods, because it is very possible that you might succumb in a moment of weakness and later, of course, regret your action.

Refrain from eating processed foods. Most people who consume these types of food gradually put on weight and have major health problems. Pay a lot of attention to how meals are prepared in your home, too, using pure, good quality ingredients. By cooking the simple recipes in the Slimmer nutrition program, you can see and know what you are putting in your body. The difference between fresh, homemade food and processed food is like the difference between night and day!

> Always keep in mind that you should choose
> quality instead of quantity.

Learn to make quality your passion! For example, a first-class quality piece of dark chocolate can be such a delicious treat and is a far cry from traditional candy bars that contain chemical preservatives and artificial flavors.

Learn to replace junk food with "treats" of high quality that will give you a real taste sensation. Invest in the best quality, because quality always wins.

SLIMMER = POSITIVE LIVING

CONCLUSION

Until Now . . .

You used to constantly think that you were obese. You were upset at the conditions in which you lived; you always talked and thought about it, repeating how destructive obesity was for you and claimed that once and for all, you had to do something to rid yourself of your excess pounds. In other words, you were completely preoccupied with your obesity and focused persistently on your great need to lose weight.

But from Now On . . .

· Keep your focus on Slimmer. Think about it constantly and visualize the slim figure you will get with its help.

· Begin to use the nutritional program right now, cooking the Slimmer way, and choosing sweet treats from Happy Moments. Now is the time for action.

· Read the psychological texts daily without fail.

· Note your thoughts in the book. You can even draw in it, making it your own!

· Talk about Slimmer with your workmates, your friends, family, and everybody.

· Think positively, think of the solution (Slimmer), feel good, and act.

To change a situation—in this case, obesity—you must not focus on the problem—that is, your excess body weight and your need to reduce it.

Focus instead on the solution—the Slimmer nutrition system—and the expected result: your own ideal weight.

As a final exercise:

Imagine that there are three black and white bubbles over your head, like the ones in the comics, with three different images of yourself. The first bubble is you at the weight you are today; the second an image of you at an even greater weight; and the third is of you at your own ideal weight. Separate the third bubble and get rid of the other two. Always keep it above your head in your imagination as a companion to whatever you do. Concentrate on it and focus your thoughts on the image of your body at your ideal weight. Because only when you are at your own ideal weight in your mind will you be able to do what you need to do—to faithfully apply the Slimmer nutritional program so that you can have the slim body you have always wanted.

Index

About the Author

Harry Papas was born in Athens, Greece. At the age of 19, and at 280 pounds, he decided it was crucial that he find a solution to his weight problem. He studied at the Department of Dietetics of the Harokopio University of Athens, Greece, and acquired his Bachelor's Degree in 1998. Along with his studies, personal experience with health and diet issues led Papas to create Slimmer, his own diet plan—and his success was remarkable. This unique program helped him regain his health, lose weight, and remain slim.

After successfully passing the exam from the Greek Ministry of Health, he became a registered dietitian in Greece and the rest of the European Union countries. He established his own Health and Diet Centre in Athens. The success of this center was unprecedented, as thousands of overweight Greek people finally found the solution to their excess weight problems by following and adopting the Slimmer program.

The next step for Papas was to incorporate his successful nutrition program into a book to help as many people as possible. *Slimmer* immediately became the most successful and bestselling diet and health book ever published in Greece.